Steady

Steady

*A Guide to Better Mental Health
Through and Beyond the Coronavirus
Pandemic*

Dr Sarb Johal

Act as if what you do makes a difference. It does.

— William James

Contents

Introduction

On the first day of my clinical psychology training at University College London in 2000, Course Co-Director, Professor Tony Roth came into the training teaching room to address the new students.

What he said that day perfectly encapsulated what I had already learned in the preceding 10 years as a psychologist, and what I have continued to experience in the years since, whether one-on-one working with clients in clinical practice, advising government and ministers, or sharing insights through the media.

His words resonated so strongly with me that they have become my core professional belief:

The central task of a psychologist is to help people live with uncertainty.

Uncertainty can show itself in so many ways. The precarious existence of so many people all around the world means that they find it difficult to plan even more than a few days ahead. Sometimes even that may feel like a very long time, fraught with tough decisions on how to spend what little money they may have and how to pay for rent, food, transport and healthcare.

For others, it can show itself as existential dread. We all have an illusory cocoon of invulnerability that enables us to get on with everyday living despite the risks we must take every day. Yet in one moment that cocoon can be punctured, revealing the fragility of life and the seemingly futile ways in which we attempt to ward off the inevitable consequence of our death. This can bring on a re-examination of life's purpose and meaning, which can be hard to deal with in times when we are reminded of our vulnerability each day.

For many of us, the Covid-19 pandemic has activated this uncertainty and anxiety. At the start of 2020, few of us could have predicted the way the virus would sweep the globe, fundamentally changing almost every aspect of our daily lives. Freedoms we took for granted — spending time with loved ones, leaving the house at will, going to church or a sports game, carefree supermarket shopping — disappeared overnight.

At first, you may have thought going into lockdown was the hard part. *Let's just get through the next four weeks, stamp out the virus and things will get back to some sort of normal.*

Now we know from experiences all over the world, that it doesn't work like that. We can stay home for a time, we can throw up strict border controls while we wait for a vaccine and treatments to be developed, yet still find ourselves locked in a cycle of escalating case numbers all over again.

The lasting economic impacts of Covid-19 and the public health measures enacted to contain its spread and protect the most vulnerable are substantial and only starting to make themselves felt. Work has changed and will continue to require substantial adjustment or even realignment. People have lost jobs with no way of knowing whether work will ever return in that form. Opportunities for other employment have dried up, with competition for jobs becoming even fiercer than it was before. Existing relationships are under strain, as people struggle to deal with the practical problems of being required to stay home in perhaps cramped and difficult living circumstances.

For those that have jobs, 'working from home' has become a completely different scenario when compared to pre-Covid times. Where once you might have worked at home for a day to complete a difficult task in peace and quiet, working from home in the middle of a global pandemic, while simultaneously running a household and acting as schoolteacher, is a completely different proposition.

Depending on current restrictions wherever you may live, even just leaving the house for work or to get groceries can take serious planning, to keep ourselves and our loved ones safe. To make matters worse, the rising tide of disinformation and the politicisation of public health measures designed to keep the public safe have contributed to a worsening sense of uncertainty. Many people have experienced leadership as lacking and have been left feeling ill-prepared to cope with whatever comes next.

At an international level, it's clear that the terms of reference for travel and trade have fundamentally changed. What this will look like and how long this will last is difficult to know, but in New Zealand, the government's Treasury department has predicted that the borders to international travellers are likely to remain closed until early 2022. It's worth noting that although the advent of viable vaccine candidates likely to be available as early as December 2020 may change this, the practical challenges of being able to vaccinate everyone who needs or wants it remains. Vaccine hesitancy and deliberate misinformation campaigns may temper uptake of the vaccine, meaning that the pandemic may not peter out quite as quickly as the more optimistic projections in recent weeks.

Demand for goods and trade across international borders and regions is changing, perhaps in a lasting way. It's possible that manufacturing bases and supply chains will be reshaped to provide better resilience against future similar shocks. This could mean significant changes to working practices and incomes for parts of the world that have in recent years become workshops serving globalised demand. Indeed, this could signal the end of times for globalisation as we currently know it. Many economic and wider strategic plans are noticeably silent concerning the 2020–2022 period. It's just too difficult to forecast, with so many variables at play.

None of this becomes clearer until effective vaccines become widely available and so the development of a vaccine has become the holy grail for many different pharmaceutical companies, supported by massive funding from governments across the world. This seems to have paid dividends, with vaccine trial data indicating that effectiveness rates of up to 95% have been achieved and licences for use being issued by regulatory authorities. On the one hand, this is astonishingly encouraging. On the other, the danger of 'vaccine nationalism' and practical obstacles such as supply chains, cold storage, and capacity to actually get the vaccine into enough arms at scale means that the ability of vaccines to truly tackle the coronavirus in a global way could be fraught with difficulty. This in turn means that the pandemic may continue on for longer than it might otherwise. Global cooperation and coordination on these issues has been sadly lacking, despite the best efforts of the World Health Organization.

If all of this sounds a bit depressing, then rest assured you are not alone in feeling that way.

Faced with all this stress and uncertainty, it's hard to summon the energy required to keep on keeping on when there is no end in sight. It's difficult to return to tight restrictions if we've been fortunate enough to taste aspects of freedom again.

How do we do life — pay the bills, juggle work and homeschool, stay mentally and emotionally well amid the constant possibility of escalating restrictions — with ongoing economic uncertainty, financial difficulties and the looming threat of Covid-19?

These questions are at the heart of this book.

How this book came about

Service to humanity is a core tenet of the Sikh tradition and so I seek to serve others with the knowledge that I am privileged to hold. In early February 2020, when it became clear to me that Covid-19 was going to become a global crisis that would endure for some time, I prepared myself to apply the experience, knowledge and expertise accumulated over a 30-year career as a psychologist where it could be most useful.

My experience as a psychologist encompasses clinical practice, frontline services, policy development and ministerial advice and strategic communications, as well as sharing insights through the media. Since 2009, I've helped the New Zealand and UK governments, as well as the World Health Organization, develop psychosocial responses to some of the major crises of the last decade, including the H1N1 pandemic, the Canterbury earthquakes, the Kaikoura earthquake, the Christchurch mosque shootings and, of course, the Covid-19 pandemic.

Psychosocial resilience and recovery looks at the combined influence of psychological and social factors on an individual's physical and mental wellbeing, and their ability to function well through challenging circumstances. It's not about reaching some finish line or returning to normality. It's an ongoing process of positively adapting to a changed (or changing) reality. It aims to improve wellbeing by strengthening your capacity to handle difficult feelings and changing circumstances, caring for your physical and emotional needs, and improving your relationships and support networks.

As the Covid-19 pandemic unfolded, I resolved to use all of this knowledge and experience in psychosocial recovery and disaster response to promote good public mental health decisions and offer support wherever I could. That meant providing strategic advice to government agencies and organisations to help leaders communicate more effectively, send the right message, and support their people through this tough time.

It also meant sharing my knowledge with the public through media appearances, my blog, my YouTube channel and this book. I wanted to shine a light on what people may be experiencing and to translate complex psychological theory into simple, understandable and useful tips and tools that will help us all get through.

We are living through an event like no other in history, taking place in a globally connected world where information travels at the speed of light. Even faster than the virus.

That's also where our advantage lies: through information and behaviour. Science helps to discover the information which shapes the decisions we make to protect ourselves and others, stop the virus from spreading and safeguard our mental wellbeing along the way. It also helps develop the treatments and vaccines which we hope will deal with the virus itself.

And while we wait for treatments and vaccines to be certified as safe and to become widely available, we have our behaviour. Our behaviour remains our best tool in the box to help us adjust to the shifting demands of Covid-19 and other future crises.

So that's what this book is all about. It's about strengthening your capacity to ride the coming waves of Covid-19 — as well as life's general ups and downs — with more calm, ease and a sense of groundedness. I share tools, tips and resources I have developed based on principles of psychosocial recovery, knowledge gained in supporting others through prolonged crises, and lessons learned during the first waves of Covid-19.

Together, this knowledge provides a framework for structuring our behaviour and our lives to support ourselves, our communities and the most vulnerable, so we can live well even with the ongoing uncertainty of Covid-19.

Living in New Zealand, I acknowledge that I have been privileged to have watched this pandemic unfold from a relatively calm place, free of the mass outbreaks and political turmoil unfolding elsewhere in the world. Nonetheless, the principles I share are evidence-based and can be applied in any crisis and in any situation. No matter how difficult your personal circumstances, getting proactive about your psychological wellbeing will help you manage your mental health, so you can keep your equilibrium and sense of wellbeing even in the midst of all of this ongoing change.

The journey has been tough and the path remains uncertain. We don't know exactly how things are going to play out, but we do know that seas are likely to be choppy. The tips and tools I share in this book will help you feel like you are standing on dry land, even if it feels like the water is rising around you, and to maintain your steadiness; to anchor you at times when you can't see the shoreline.

The better we care for ourselves and others, the more likely it is that we will come through this difficult time intact, healthy and ready to face the future. Together.

So let's begin.

Sarb

CHAPTER 1

The trouble with uncertainty

Human beings are creatures of habit. We like predictability and routine, so our everyday lives tend to follow a familiar pattern: We go to work, we go to the gym, we take the kids to after-school activities, we eat dinner, we watch our favourite TV shows, we go to bed. On the weekend we might play or watch sport, do a little DIY, catch up with friends, sleep late or attend a religious service.

In 'normal' times, this predictability helps most of us to navigate everyday life on a fairly even keel. With our neat weekly schedules in place, we usually know what's happening next, so we tend not to worry too much about what's around the corner. This sense of continuity gives meaning to our lives and allows us to believe that the world is a safe, stable and generally positive place — or at least, not a place that is likely to cause us harm.

The trouble is, those 'normal times' seemed to evaporate somewhere around March 2020, when the Covid-19 pandemic began rapidly spreading across the globe.

We humans are used to dealing with viruses. Seasonal flu happens every year and while we know that it can be deadly for some, it's also a familiar threat, with some predictability. Plus we have vaccines and medications to protect the most vulnerable, so we can prepare ahead of time for flu season.

In contrast, Covid-19 seemed to spring out of nowhere, quickly taking hold and causing chaotic and frightening scenes in hospitals from Wuhan to Milan and New York City. To make matters worse, Covid-19 came loaded with uncertainty. *Who is at risk? Who can spread it and how? What protective steps should I take? How effective will the treatments be? How will the outbreak unfold? When can we travel or see our loved ones again? Will there be another wave? Is it safe to send my kids to school?*

Uncertainty is recognised as a leading cause of worry, anxiety and stress. When we don't know what's coming next, we feel vulnerable and this puts us on edge. This edginess is exacerbated when official advice seems to be conflicting or constantly changing, as knowledge of the virus unfolds or official bodies offer differing opinions.

The unfamiliarity of Covid-19 combined with the sudden extreme uncertainty of our everyday lives when faced with unprecedented lockdowns and restrictions, ramped up our anxiety levels, putting us on high alert. This response makes sense when you think of it as an evolutionary legacy: in the face of an unfamiliar risk, erring on the side of caution may be a better way to survive, rather than assuming everything will be fine.

On the downside, all this change can feel like a whirlwind, leaving you churned up inside, feeling anxious, worried, and even frightened about the future. Contrast this with our usual craving for predictability and routine, and it's no surprise that many of us find the ongoing uncertainty of Covid-19 more difficult than definitively knowing that something bad is going to happen.

So how can you tell if all this uncertainty is throwing you out of kilter?

In an acute or prolonged crisis, most people will experience some distress in the form of difficult feelings and emotions. Take a moment to reflect and consider whether you or your loved ones have experienced any of the following since the onset of this pandemic:

- Stress or overwhelm
- Anxiety, worry, or fear
- Sadness, tearfulness, and/or loss of interest in usual enjoyable activities
- Physical symptoms, such as increased heart rate, stomach upset, low energy, or other uncomfortable sensations
- Frustration, irritability, or anger
- Helplessness
- Difficulty concentrating or sleeping
- Isolating or withdrawing from others, and/or fear of going to public spaces.

If you said 'yes' to one or more of these experiences, you are not alone. These are all common reactions in situations that are uncertain and evolving. And just because you're feeling okay one day, doesn't automatically mean that you're going to feel okay the next. You might find yourself feeling a bit up and down, or perhaps progressively more flat. All of this is normal — we are living through an extraordinary time.

The good news is that your emotions, including anxiety, are there for a reason. They carry messages and alert us to situations that we need to address. They can also motivate us into action.

That's when our anxiety is working for us. But sometimes it works against us. Instead of motivating us to act, it can be paralysing and cause us to feel overwhelmed or shut down.

To understand how our emotions can work for us and against us, we need to understand the three internal systems that govern our everyday behaviour: the threat system, the calming system, and the drive or motivation system.

The **threat system** is the basic smoke detector in your brain. This system alerts you when danger is detected and you need to be concerned, watch out or take action.

Threat detection is a complex process involving the whole brain and, more specifically, the limbic system. This system is a set of structures in the brain that deals with emotions and memory. It also governs our fight, flight and freeze behaviours.

Once activated, the threat system concentrates your attention and resources on doing something about the threat. It's designed to save your life, by alerting you of the need to get out of danger immediately.

The threat system automatically fires up your sympathetic nervous system, which acts like an accelerator, preparing the body for 'fight or flight'. It floods the body with hormones and sharpens your alertness and your senses, so that you can see and hear more clearly and make better sense of what is happening around you. It accelerates the heart rate and moves blood flow away from processes like digesting food, towards your muscles, so that you can strike back or get the heck out of that dangerous situation.

These processes are supposed to be temporary, lasting just long enough for us to be out of danger and safe again. This also explains why we like to drink coffee and other stimulants, as the acceleration can help us to focus in the short term.

Sometimes, though, the 'fight or flight' response can lead to paralysis. This is an evolutionary hangover, because we may have been predated upon by creatures that had extremely sensitive movement receptors in their eyes. Staying still can trick these predators into thinking there is nothing there to attack, because they aren't detecting any movement. This explains why you see animals 'frozen in the headlights' when crossing roads.

In this age of the pandemic, the ongoing unpredictability and uncertainty keeps your threat detection system firing a lot of the time. This is especially the case if you're checking the news a lot, or spending a lot of time thinking or worrying about the pandemic. The more time you spend looking at information that your brain finds threatening, like 24-hour news channels or doom-scrolling on your phone, the more you stoke the threat detection response. Your brain responds as if your life is at risk, even when that's not true in the moment.

When your brain is constantly responding as if you are in imminent danger, it's very hard to do anything else. Your brain is focused on staying alive and you simply don't have the mental space or resources necessary for creative problem-solving and strategic thinking. These activities that are so crucial in a crisis get demoted to 'nice-to-have-once-I-survive-this-threat' status. Your brain doesn't particularly care where you're headed, it just wants to deal with the threat — and it's exhausting.

If you allow yourself to stay in threat mode the whole time, your brain creates shortcuts for dealing with stress and staying alive. You end up repeating these shortcuts without any conscious control, which will most likely end up less than optimal for you in the long term.

The key to bringing our creativity and strategic thinking back online lies in learning to intentionally calm ourselves. If the sympathetic nervous system acts like the accelerator in your car, then the parasympathetic nervous system is your brake. This **calming system** brings your body back to equilibrium after a stressful situation, slowing your breathing and your heart rate, bringing digestive activity back, and relaxing your muscles.

You can activate your calming, parasympathetic nervous system by doing activities like deep belly-breathing. This calming activity presses the brake and eases the pressure on the threat detection system. The threat detection system senses that the internal environment is changing, and eases back on the alert levels. As your alert levels drop, you can begin to devote your attention and resources to things other than immediate life preservation.

That's why spending time on mastering your brake is so important. When you take intentional control of this calming system, you're no longer driven by threat. It tells your brain that there is no need to limit your capacity to solving this life-threatening situation, so you are then free to do other things.

The third system is your **drive or motivation system**. Once you're able to use that accelerator and brake more smoothly, you need to know where you're headed, right?

But what if your life destination looks completely different to where you were headed before the pandemic struck? You may think that you need the equivalent of a GPS navigation system in your brain to guide your behaviour. But a GPS can get confused if you lose signal, or if it hasn't been updated as the terrain of the world changes around you in these unpredictable and uncertain times.

What you really need is something more basic: a compass. And the best compass to help steer you through troubled waters and uncharted territory is your value system.

We'll talk more about your values and how to define them in chapter 13. For now, simply note that your motivation or drive system cannot be fully expressed when your foot is jammed on the accelerator. When you're constantly revving the engine higher and higher trying to escape a threat, you can't live in alignment with your values or get to where you really want to go.

That's why it's so important to learn how to intentionally activate your calming system. When you can consciously choose to apply the brake, you can bring your body out of threat and back to an equilibrium. This allows your drive system to kick in, so you can take back a little control over your direction and move forward towards the things that really matter to you.

The antidote to uncertainty

It's clear that we are going to have to live with the uncertainty of Covid-19 for some time, most likely until effective vaccines are confirmed as safe and taken up widely, and treatment becomes readily available.

Facing this particular brand of uncertainty is hard. The ground seems to be constantly shifting beneath us, the usual settings of our lives are disrupted and there's no firm endpoint in sight. Meanwhile, the pressures and stresses of life continue, or may even have been augmented by the times. Most of us still need to work, take care of family members or fulfil community obligations. Some of us will need to add in homeschooling, financial stress, or health worries. Life goes on, even if the form has altered.

If we don't have the option (or the desire) to hibernate until the threat of Covid-19 has passed, then our only choice is to keep on doing life as best we can. That's why the most effective way to come through this pandemic with our wellbeing intact is to adjust our behaviour to meet the demands of the time. That means learning to consciously influence our three internal systems, so we can live well, safeguard our wellbeing, and continue to find joy and satisfaction even when we don't know what's around the corner.

When we learn to disengage our threat system, we are no longer at the mercy of worry and uncertainty and we don't have to operate as if our lives are constantly in danger. We can then start to pay attention to the broader structure of our lives, reducing our anxiety and uncertainty.

As we consciously engage our calming system, we can access the more creative and strategic facets of our minds to bring new solutions to bear — solutions which we do not have the capacity to generate when we are frightened and dominated by uncertainty.

As we begin to regain control, we can access our drive system, find our motivation and direction, and begin to develop the skills to live well alongside uncertainty. Hope returns and we begin to entertain future possibilities that do not automatically fill us with existential dread.

As we learn to manage our internal systems well, there are two more factors that come into play: **structure and empathy**. Structure — such as rules, routines or guidelines — can help us manage uncertainty, while empathy helps us accept and adapt to the structure, or smooths the path when structure alone is not enough. The psychological literature, and my personal experience supporting people through acute and prolonged periods of crisis, has taught me that people need a balance of both in order to stay well and perform well in uncertain environments.

This is also where we may need external assistance. Governments, leaders and organisations can help us get through difficult times, by providing clear structures to help us navigate our daily reality, and delivering those structures with empathy for people's lived experiences. We'll dive deeper into structure and empathy, and how they can help you live well with uncertainty, in the next chapters.

Throughout this book, you'll find tools and techniques to influence your three internal systems of threat, calm, and drive, so you can navigate life on a more even keel no matter what may come. That's not to say that any of this is easy. It takes consistency, practice and flexibility to fully reap the benefits. But in a time when so much is out of our control, these tools will help you stay on track.

The better you become at managing your internal states, the more likely it is that you will not only survive, but thrive through this pandemic and beyond.

CHAPTER 2

Structure

In an unexpected or prolonged crisis, people crave structure. Even the smallest elements of structure can restore some sense of order, predictability and safety to our world. It gives us something to hold on to and helps us to feel like we do have a tiny bit of control, even if the world as we know it has been turned upside down.

We can create structure for ourselves, through healthy routines and boundaries. When all around us is uncertain and is making us feel afraid, we can organise our lives to make sure we do the things that make us feel better, and that we don't expose ourselves to things that make us feel worse. Structure also acts like a container, helping us put boundaries around our anxiety so that it doesn't spill out and colour the entire day. It helps us to be intentional about the way we use our time, so that we can see whether we are living in alignment with our values (or not) and maintain our equilibrium, even though we may be worried or feeling low.

Sometimes, though, circumstances will be so challenging that either we can't create our own structure, or we find it hard to think of a structure that will keep us focused. That's when it can help to look to others. We can seek guidance from those around us, to help us build realistic routines so we can get things done, manage our anxiety and start to rebuild our lives in ways that will keep our loved ones safe, fed, housed and out of economic ruin.

To get through a crisis well, we must work in partnership with our loved ones and our communities, but we also need clear leadership from the government and other authorities. They can provide us with structure to help us manage all the things we need to do in order to keep ourselves well and safe. These structures could take the form of laws, guidelines, advice, or financial and emotional support schemes.

Good structures will be well thought out, clearly defined and helpful, rather than kneejerk responses to the latest threat. It's a fine balance though, because while good structure is essential, too much structure can make us feel stifled, especially when it's imposed upon us. That's where empathy comes in. We need our leaders to help us understand what is being asked of us, why it is being asked, and, so far as possible, how it might impact us in the future, so that we can connect to our personal internal drive system and find the motivation to do what we need to do. Essentially, people want to know what to do, whether or not they are doing it correctly, and if their actions are having an impact.

We'll talk more about how governments can provide helpful structure and communicate effectively in chapter 7.

Creating everyday structure

How can you put in place everyday structures that will support your individual wellbeing in uncertain times?

The first step is to **make sure your basic resources are covered**. There are things that you need to live your life, like money, food, shelter and access to good information. It's important to ask for support if these are lacking for you. Many governments have rolled out specific support packages for businesses and individuals as a result of the pandemic, so if you're struggling, find out what is available and whether you are eligible.

Next, **take care of your health**. Adopting precautionary behaviours can help you feel reassured and secure, so keep up the everyday precautions, washing your hands often and thoroughly with soap and water, especially before you eat, or using hand sanitiser if you can't get to soap and water. These are good habits for life, not just for Covid-19. Of course we've known this since we were children, but some of us have learned that we weren't taking enough care with these simple tasks, like washing for long enough, or getting soap into all the little nooks and crannies.

Follow official advice designed to keep you safe, such as advice regarding the wearing of masks and congregating in groups (especially when indoors). Using a Covid-19 tracer app or other technological aid where you live will help with contact tracing in the event of an outbreak, or you can keep a diary if you don't feel comfortable with an app or other technology.

If you need to stay at home, or if you are feeling unwell, remember that social distancing actually means physical distancing. Stay away from others physically, but remember to reach out and connect with others however you can.

Third, think about your routine. If you're working from home, or trying to juggle other priorities like parenting and homeschooling, you may need to impose structures to ensure that the most important tasks get done. Remember, you'll experience less distress if you implement that structure with empathy, which means being realistic in your expectations and being kind to yourself if you've had a hard day. More on that in chapter 3.

How to work from home

If you're fortunate enough to be in a location-flexible job with ongoing work, then chances are you've found yourself working from home at least some of the time. Whether you're a seasoned veteran or a complete newbie to this work-from-home thing, it's likely to be part of your life for some time.

For many of us, **working from home** was previously considered a temporary situation. Perhaps you didn't have any face-to-face meetings booked, so you decided to avoid the office for the day. Maybe you needed a block of time without the constant interruptions from co-workers, so you brought your laptop home for the day and set it on the kitchen table.

In ordinary times, working from home represents a significant change from your normal routine and pace of work. This can be very effective once in a while, precisely because it's different from normal. You still have the usual framework and structure of your daily routine, and your colleagues in the office adjust their work in light of your absence.

Since the Covid-19 pandemic unfolded, many organisations have people working outside their offices all the time. We call this **remote working** and it requires a very different set of abilities, resources and skills. Assuming you have the space, the office perks can be incredible at home, but they can be incredibly distracting too, especially with other people or young children around.

Working remotely day after day needs a self-starting attitude and ninja-level time management skills. To get it right, you need structure, plus a shared understanding of expectations and what's going to function well for both the organisation and the person working at home. Here are some tips to get you started.

1. Do something that isn't work first. If you were working out, you'd probably stretch and warm up first. Okay, I know you don't, but you should, because otherwise you're not going to perform at your best, and you might get hurt and you'll be sore for days.

The same is true for work. Start your day by warming up your brain with a non-work task. Go for a walk, listen to a podcast, or exercise. And no, checking your email doesn't count, because this flips your mind into work mode (even if they are non-work emails). It's best to stay off any interface that signals to your brain that work is about to begin.

2. Chunk your time. One of the great things about remote work is that you don't have to show up at 8am and stay till 5pm. One of the worst things about remote work is that you don't have to show up at 8am and stay till 5pm, and there are so many distractions competing for your time. If you're not careful, time can slip away and you end up staying up late just to get your regular tasks done.

Block your time, and give each block of time a purpose: email, writing, research or meetings. This makes it easier to control your flow of work, handle interruptions when they come, and get back on task when you engage again.

Check out the Pomodoro Technique for one way of chunking your time into 25-minute blocks of focused work, each followed by a five-minute break. Many people find this a helpful way of concentrating their work activity into highly productive blocks, followed by a short break when they can move around, do some stretches, make a cuppa or pop the washing machine on. Try using the Pomodoro Technique to set a goal of completing a task you have been avoiding — you'll be amazed by how much you can get done in 25 minutes when you are focused.

3. Turn off notifications. Nothing kills productivity like incoming notifications. Turn them off, and then set a reminder to check your emails three times a day: at the start of the day, just before lunch, and once more just before you finish your scheduled working day. Don't get sucked into the email vortex that kills many hours for even the most productive of remote workers. It helps to let your colleagues know that this is how you will be working — tell them that if something requires urgent attention, they will need to pick up the phone.

4. Create your place. Create a workspace where you can focus with the minimum distractions. Even if you like to mix it up and work in different places around the house, it's important that you have somewhere you can go to concentrate and get things done, even if it's a corner of your bedroom. It also helps you define the boundary between work and home.

5. Get out in the world when you can. If you're spending too long staring at a screen or reading sheets of paper, then change your focus by looking out the window every now and again. Get up and move around in between your chunks of allocated work time, or go for a walk around the block. All this will help you be more productive, and feel more balanced. Even when you're self-isolating or in lockdown, it's important for your own state of mind to recognise that in most situations you can get outside to take some fresh air.

6. Shut the door. One of the hardest things about remote working is that sometimes I have to say 'no' to the people I love, because I have to get work done. Take time to create the expectation that when you're working, you're not going to be available for piggy-back rides, or gaming sessions with your kids. My family knows that when the door is shut, it's work time. Ask your partner, housemates, other adults or older kids for help with this too. Treat it as if you've left the house and gone to work elsewhere, knowing you'll be home at the end of the day and there will be plenty of time for piggy-backs then.

7. Dress for work. Yes, you could work in your pyjamas. But if you change and put work clothes on, you're much more likely to make the mental shift into work mode, and then stick to a work-mode structure. Staying in your slouching-around clothes makes it all too easy to blur the lines, and suddenly, you're cleaning parts of the house you never knew needed cleaning, or making that cold-brew coffee you've always thought would be amazing. Get dressed at the start of the day, and get out of your work clothes when you've finished working. Your attitude goes with the clothes.

8. Know when your day is going to end. It's tempting to let your structure slip and end up working far longer into the day than you intended to. If this continues, it's not likely to be particularly good for you, or those around you. You're far more likely to be more productive when you know your time is limited, so set a time to finish working and stick to it.

9. Remote working can be really lonely. Tell someone about your day — what you're working on and what you got done. You're more likely to be productive when you know you're going to be accountable to someone else.

10. Share the load with your partner. This is great if you have a partner around, and they live with you, or are allowed to form a bubble with you in pandemic times. You can divide the day into shifts of three hours long perhaps, and take turns working and being with the kids. But what if you don't have a partner? Well, the advice offered by parents in this situation includes radical honesty with your workplace — if you have a job that offers that kind of flexibility — and with your kids too. Let your work know in advance if you're going to do the school run, or have to start the routine of getting your kids to bed at 4.30pm (yes, it can take that long — at least, in my home with three young girls). But keeping your child or children informed of the situation is important too. If they're used to having your attention when you're home, then your working and not being able to give them that kind of attention will take some getting used to. And that's why you'll also probably need a supersized helping of structure too. If your children are still able to go to school, set key tasks to get done in the hours you'll have between drop-off and pick-up and then save jobs like admin and emails for after bedtime. If the kids are off school, set up a routine that works for you, whether it's an hour of play all together to start the day, then an hour of work for you and an hour of study/solo play or a movie for the kids followed by snack time all together, etc. Routines help kids feel safe, and they'll help you with some predictability in your day too.

In case you didn't know, kids can be noisy. And not just the small ones. So, if you're a boss and you see or hear kids in the background of Zoom calls, then have a heart. Often, the best plans go awry and parents really are trying to manage what feels like, and sometimes are, impossible situations on a day-to-day basis. Hopefully, it's not like that all the time. But it will happen.

Bonus tip: Write yourself an email at the end of the day listing everything that you managed to get done, from completed tasks to phone calls and any positive feedback you received. Send it to yourself and store these in a folder in your email service. Writing the email will capture your progress and help you focus your thoughts at the end of the day. Reading it back later will help to motivate you, as you can see what you've achieved.

The Five Ways to Wellbeing

So now we've seen how structure can help us to ensure our basic needs are covered and how it can help us work productively from home.

But structure isn't just about ticking off jobs, chores and obligations. We can use structure to enhance our wellbeing in difficult times by prioritising activities which support our physical, mental and emotional health.

One useful framework is the Five Ways to Wellbeing. These are five simple actions you can do every day to boost your mental health, pick up your energy or pull yourself out of a rut. They don't cost anything but the rewards can be priceless. When done regularly, the Five Ways are scientifically[1] proven to lift your everyday wellbeing.

The Five Ways are:

1. **Connect.** Psychological literature shows that the biggest protector in times of emergency and crisis is social connection. Staying connected helps us to feel cared for and part of a supportive social network, so it's important that we do everything we can to stay in touch with the people we know and love. Remember, social distancing really means physical distancing. If your movements are currently restricted, make an effort to find ways to connect with others, either online or by picking up the phone. Even in lockdown, you can still talk to your neighbour over the fence or say 'hi' to people on your walk, provided that you stay an appropriate distance away and/or wear a mask.

2. **Give.** Doing something nice for a friend or stranger gives a lovely boost to both the giver and the receiver. It could be as simple as paying a compliment, saying thank you, or volunteering your time for a worthy cause. Make giving a regular part of your day, and you'll find it brings incredible

1. Aked, J, Marks, N, Cordon, C, & Thompson, S (2008). Five Ways to Wellbeing: A report presented to the Foresight Project on communicating the evidence base for improving people's well-being. Centre for Well-being. The New Economics Foundation.

rewards, from unexpected conversations to new friendships, or a renewed sense of purpose. When your wellbeing becomes linked to that of your community, you'll feel an even deeper sense of connection and belonging.

3. **Notice.** One of the best ways to activate your internal brake or calming system is to practise mindfulness. This means slowing down, savouring the moment and becoming aware of what is happening all around you. Use all five senses: what can you see, touch, taste, smell and hear? There is joy in simple things, if only we pause long enough to notice.

4. **Learn.** Consciously seek out new experiences, like trying a new class (in-person or online), cooking a new recipe, reading a book in a different genre or listening to the stories and experiences of people from different backgrounds. Set a challenge that you will enjoy mastering and do a little bit each day. YouTube is full of how-to videos on everything from changing a bike tyre or planting a veggie garden to learning instruments and foreign languages. Learning something new will give your confidence a boost, bring you satisfaction and give you something new to talk about with friends and loved ones, even if you're in isolation.

5. **Stay active.** Exercise is proven to improve your mood but you don't need to buy expensive equipment or sweat it out doing burpees and push-ups unless you want to — and if you do, that's great! The key is finding an activity that you enjoy and making it part of your day, like brushing your teeth. Step outside and go for a walk or a bike ride, turn up the music and dance or get in the garden and dig. Focus on making movement fun, notice how great you feel when you're done and you will want to exercise again tomorrow.

It might help to think of these Five Ways as the mental health equivalent of the 5 a day fruit and veggie rule. At the beginning of each day, make a plan for how you can tick off as many of the five as you can. Review your list at the end of the day, and see how many you managed to complete.

Remember to approach this list with empathy for yourself and others. If you had a busy day and you didn't manage to learn something new, make a plan to do so tomorrow, or by the end of the week. If it's almost bedtime and you haven't managed to really connect with someone, take five minutes to snuggle with your child or your partner and be fully present in the moment. If you live alone, you can send a kind and thoughtful message to a friend before you go to sleep. Even a few calming yoga stretches before bed will make a difference — just make sure you also fit in longer periods of exercise across the week.

An exercise in mindful breathing

One of the best ways to activate your internal calming system or brake is through mindful breathing. The principles of mindfulness are really very simple — stop, calm, rest, notice — but the results can be profound. Here's how to get started.

Stop for a moment. Sit in silence. Breathe.

Take deep breaths in, and very slow breaths out.

If your eyes are open, try to take in the details of what you might see out your window.

What trees are swishing around outside? What colour are the cars parked outside?

Can you hear any birds? What do they sound like?

Now close your eyes and focus on the temperature of the air on your palms.

Feel the chair against your body, or your feet on the floor.

What you're doing here isn't just summoning some abstract form of inner peace. You're healing your body and your brain.

When your brain is in panic mode, flooding your system with an excess of stress hormones, these chemicals can affect your physical health by lowering your immunity, causing inflammation and even changing structures in your brain. Pulling your brain out of panic mode keeps your body operating at its best.

Mindfulness also helps you turn down the dial on the default mode network (DMN), the part of your brain that causes racing, anxious, self-conscious thoughts. The DMN is internally focused and can't operate as well when you're focusing really intently on external stimuli, without a story attached. In other words, your self-conscious head-babble tends to disappear if you're able to focus on the present, like the sensory feeling of a breeze on your face.

So, switch down the chatter of your default mode network and pay attention to what you can sense outside of you by making mindfulness a regular part of your day.

With regular practice, mindfulness will help you feel calmer, more present and more connected to the world around you. It will also give you a break from your worries and help you put them in perspective, so they don't completely take over your day.

And the best part is it's free and it doesn't have to take a lot of time. Try setting a reminder on your phone, or using your Pomodoro breaks to take 10 mindful breaths at least once an hour.

The bonus four

Once you've got your Five Ways to Wellbeing sorted, I recommend you add another four:

Relax. Take time to chill and give your mind and body a break. Take a long bath, read a book, or lie in the sun.

Eat well. We all know about the benefits of healthy eating, so make an effort to feed your brain and body well. Making a conscious effort to include nutritious, energy-rich foods will really help to lift your mood and your energy. Instead of trying to go on a diet or cut out certain food groups when you're already under stress, why not try adding things in? Toss in some greens with your scrambled eggs, have a salad at lunchtime or whip up a smoothie. By adding in extra, good stuff, you'll naturally start to crowd out the junk. That's the theory, anyway.

Get enough sleep. Good sleep is vital, particularly in stressful times. You need adequate rest in order to stay well emotionally, mentally and physically. Try sticking to a set bedtime, and keep your bedroom only for sleeping — no watching Netflix or scrolling social media in bed. (For more tips on getting a good night's sleep, check out chapter 9.)

Have fun. In tough times, it's easy to let go of the things that bring us pleasure and joy. When life is stressful, it's easy to dismiss 'fun' as superfluous, a nice-to-have rather than an essential. But pleasurable activities can help enormously to ease depressive feelings, so I recommend you add five doses of fun to every single day. It could be playing a game with your kids, listening to a comedy podcast from pre-coronavirus times, grabbing your bike and going for a fast ride or anything that makes you feel alive.

This list might seem long, but remember, these are good habits for life and they don't have to take a lot of time. Every little thing you can do to support your wellbeing will make the situation feel a little brighter and help you get through this time in better shape.

Keeping structure in lockdown

Structure is especially important when you're in lockdown, quarantine, isolation or even on holiday, when it's easy to lose track of the days.

As always, make sure your basic resources are covered, ask for help if you need it and be considerate of others' needs too, particularly if there is a shortage of testing or medical appointments, long waits at the supermarket, or you feel tempted to book up delivery slots 'just in case'.

It's also important to pay attention to what is happening around you and check advice about how to keep yourself and your loved ones safe, but try not to stray into information overload. Set a limit on how many times a day you check the news or go on social media.

Once these basics are taken care of, it helps to occupy everyone in the household with a good mix of fun, purposeful and restorative activities. Having a healthy routine, eating well, getting exercise and sleep can have a positive impact on your thoughts and feelings. If you're feeling down or depressed, you might tend to be less active than normal. You stop doing things that lift your spirits and this can be a vicious cycle that makes you feel even worse.

Whatever your current circumstances, you can use structure to bring some wellbeing and fun back into your week, by giving each day a theme from the Five Ways to Wellbeing:

- **Connection Mondays.** Make a special effort to reach out to others. And don't just send a message — pick up the phone, or get on that group chat with people that you want to talk to and fuel that connection.
- **Active Tuesdays.** If restrictions allow, step outside and play a game, garden, cycle, walk or run. Try a physical activity that is new to you and suits your level of mobility and fitness.
- **Mindful Wednesdays** are all about taking notice and being curious. Observe the beauty all around us. Watch the weather through the window as it changes. Notice how the seasons are changing. Remark on the unusual. Savour your coffee and your food. Be aware of what you are feeling, hearing and seeing in the world around you.
- **Teach me Thursdays.** Make learning the key focus for the day. Try something new, rediscover an old pastime, try a new recipe, or set a challenge that you'll enjoy achieving. Do it on your own, with others in your household or online with friends.
- **Giving Fridays.** Fridays are all about giving, so try some

random acts of kindness by doing something nice for someone else. Send a thank you note or a video message, check in on a neighbour or try to help someone out online.

Having simple and nourishing structure to the week helps you organise your time and creates a purposeful focus for each day, not just for you, but for family and especially your kids.

Another way to create structure in lockdown is by incorporating simple yet fun daily rituals. In the bustle of daily life, it's easy to pass each other by. Taking time together each day to do something with shared meaning has the effect of slowing us down and creating an opportunity to connect. Something as simple as sharing a family or community meal can have a profound impact on wellbeing and connection. By making a safe space and a regular routine of coming together to share our experiences, we can learn from each other, create deeper mutual understanding, and express our personal or cultural values and traditions.

In times of stress, it's even more important to remember to turn towards each other. Rituals can help us to process our feelings and stay connected despite our conflicts. When we disagree, experience conflict, or there is a threat with the potential to tear communities apart, we can turn away from each other, inwardly stewing or seeking refuge in people who reinforce our polarised position.

Rituals that bring us together begin the process of repair. By creating repeated opportunities to come together, rituals help us maintain these connections. They offer opportunities to iron out differences and maintain closeness, rather than diverging into our personal echo chambers.

The best part is, rituals don't have to be formal or serious to make a difference. If you're stuck in lockdown, or even if you're not, here are a few fun and not-serious rituals you can bring into your day to add meaning, laughter and build connection with others.

1. Write down one thing you wanted to say yesterday, but didn't. This one is best done first thing in the morning. The days can blend into each other if you're not careful. Things can be said in haste for sure, but sometimes we can fail to say things that, on reflection, we wish we had. This ritual gives you the opportunity to revisit yesterday in a way that breaks a pattern of what you did; instead, it helps you to focus on something that you didn't do, but wanted to. That then becomes something you can tackle today.

2. Write a do-not-do list. Jot down things you did today that are not really helping. Tomorrow, see if you can replace them with habits and activities that support your wellbeing. Do this ritual regularly, and over time you'll crowd out the unhelpful stuff and bring in more of the good stuff.

3. Make a graffiti board. Find one large piece of paper and tag it every day, any way you like, and perhaps invite others to join in too. See what emerges over time and how your feelings, mood or experiences are reflected in your tags. You can find ways to do this online too.

4. Draw a mouse. Draw it every day and see how it evolves over the next few weeks. Doing the same creative (but somewhat nonsensical) task challenges you to bring some creativity to the table. But it also allows you to see how your response to the ritual changes on a daily basis. Do this together with others and you can share a laugh or moments of poignancy over what you've come up with.

5. Grab a picture from your cellphone. Every day, write the most absurd caption you can imagine for it. Choose a different photo every day.

6. Jot down the first five words that come into your head, then arrange them to tell a one-sentence story that represents your day. And yes, you can add filler words.

7 Another fun way to capture your day and make a creative record of this time is by **creating an acronym**. Take the first letter of your first name and the second letter of your last name — in my case S for Sarb and O from Johal. Re-interpret that acronym every day in a way that represents your day. For example, today might have been Silly Official, but tomorrow I might be Sad Owl, or Slightly Odd. This tool acts like a frame to record your emotions and events in a shorthand diary. Look back on it every now and again, and it's a shorthand record on how you might have been feeling at that very moment in time. It's also a creative act that forces you to use a slightly different part of your problem-solving repertoire, rather than the part of your brain that decides what you're going to have for dinner.

Good structure helps us get through uncertain times in better shape, by providing a framework to ensure we have what we need, and that we are consistently doing more of the things that nourish and less of the things that will stress or deplete. Structure also helps us to integrate calming actions and activities into everyday life, so we can hit the brake, step out of constant crisis mode and begin to move forward.

But structure can only be applied well with a healthy dose of empathy. That's what we'll explore in the next chapter.

CHAPTER 3

Empathy

For the vast majority of us, this pandemic has been way outside our normal range of experience. We haven't been trained for this and we weren't prepared for it, so it's no surprise that sometimes it can all feel more than a little overwhelming.

While we may live in the same country, or the same community, each of us will be experiencing the Covid-19 pandemic and lockdown differently within those societies. The amount of stress and pressure we might feel will depend on a number of factors including our health, our family situation, our work pressures, our financial position, any pre-existing stressors and the degree to which we feel supported and connected.

When our individual experiences of a crisis are so different, empathy becomes incredibly important. Empathy is the ability to stand in someone else's shoes, to understand what they are feeling even if we haven't had the same experience ourselves. When we feel empathy, this enables prosocial or helping behaviours to flow from within, rather than being forced. We naturally want to reach out and support others.

Even in good times, empathy is crucial for establishing healthy relationships and learning how to behave compassionately. It applies to our ability to recognise, understand and share the thoughts and feelings of not only another person, but animals and fictional characters too. That's why the way people — real or imagined — are depicted in the media is so important, because it will have an impact on how much empathy we feel for that person and their situation, and consequently our response.

Our initial bolt of empathy is automatic. It occurs when we can observe or imagine what someone else is feeling, and it triggers the same sort of feeling in us. True empathy occurs when we can be present with those feelings. We don't dismiss them or gloss over them to make ourselves feel more comfortable. We listen, acknowledge and seek to understand.

When someone listens and offers empathy, what they are really saying is 'You are not alone in feeling the way you do'. That's incredibly powerful. It makes us feel heard and understood. It normalises the struggle we might be experiencing. It eases our anxiety, helps us process tough circumstances and move through difficult emotions more quickly, so that we can take positive steps to move forward again.

We can think of empathy in many ways, but a distinction into two types can be helpful here. We think of cognitive empathy as that rational-based idea of putting yourself in someone's shoes, or 'empathy by thought', and emotional empathy as 'empathy by feelings', when you quite literally feel the other person's emotions alongside them, as if you had 'caught' the emotions.

Here's where we can get into trouble: when we experience empathy, we also feel vulnerable. When we open ourselves up to recognise difficult feelings in others, we feel or reflect upon them in ourselves too. We might feel frustration, sadness, anger or a sense of feeling stuck. It's uncomfortable, even painful, and it can bring up memories or physical sensations that we'd rather forget. If we aren't well-versed in how to manage our emotions, then empathy can overwhelm us. Instead of responding with healthy empathic concern, we respond with empathic distress.

Empathic distress is a me-focused response — empathy that turns into emotional quicksand when we just keep 'feeling with' a person (feeling and feeling and feeling) without doing anything to try to change their situation. In time, we get overwhelmed by the distress we're experiencing at their distress, and we don't know what to do with our painful feelings. This often leads to 'withdrawal behaviour', as we try to escape our uncomfortable emotions by becoming irritated, snapping at the other person, shutting down or ducking out and leaving them alone with their suffering. The discomfort makes us pull back from others when they need us most, because it's too painful to keep contact.

If you're a parent, you might find this happening with your child or teen. After listening to an outpouring of teenage angst or what might *seem* like self-indulgence, you become irritated and shut down the conversation, creating disconnection when your teen needs you most.

If this sounds familiar, be reassured that it's a common response. The good news is that we can choose to funnel our empathy in another direction, so that it becomes helpful rather than harmful. This is called **empathic concern**, where we switch the focus from trying to manage the emotion we are feeling, to trying to do something practical to help the other person.

Empathic concern is an other-focused response. Some have described it as similar to feeling moved, touched or having heart-warming feelings. It starts with our experiencing that initial bolt of 'feeling with' a person who is suffering, but then we shift into 'feeling for' — as in 'What can I do for you?'

Empathic concern is otherwise known as compassionate empathy and basically means *empathy with an action plan*, motivating us to try to make things better for another person. Moving from pain into action helps us to manage the emotion and avoid the overwhelm.

It also helps the other person move through their pain quicker and get to a better outcome.

Sometimes the action might simply be listening and being with that person, if that's what you think they need. The key is to actively listen, and to see the value of this as an action. This means making a conscious decision to listen to and understand the messages of the speaker — whether that's in the words they are saying, or something deeper. It takes work to really listen, but it's an incredibly powerful way to show that you are taking someone else's experience seriously.

The important takeaway here is that you don't have to let your feelings run the show. Instead, you can take control of your feelings by shifting from me-driven empathy and empathic distress, to empathic concern. In practice, this simply takes redirecting your focus from how upset you are, to how helpful you can be — emotionally and practically.

Your action plan doesn't have to be complicated. The items on your empathic concern to-do list will be things like calling your loved ones, sending a care package, making a blanket fort with the kids, staying home when appropriate and arranging for a neighbour to check on an isolated loved one.

If a friend is going through a difficult break-up with a boyfriend you didn't like, empathic concern might mean reserving judgement, listening attentively, giving her a hug and focusing on her feelings instead of what you think should happen next. If a co-worker has to work the weekend and you don't have the expertise to offer practical assistance and ease his workload, you might pop in on Saturday morning to deliver a coffee and a doughnut, along with a few encouraging words.

Empathy with an action plan doesn't take an empathic genius. It mostly just takes showing up, being present and reassuring others that they are not alone. Think of this as striking the balance between logic and emotion. Perhaps we have an idea about what people could do to help their situation, but we temper the temptation to become unsympathetic and irritated with their lack of action, or to be overwhelmed with our own emotions. We can feel another person's pain, as if it were happening to us, and therefore express the appropriate amount of sympathy. At the same time, we can remain in control of our own emotions, apply reason and withhold judgement. This means we can make better decisions and provide better support where they need it most.

Here are six ways that you can practise empathy with an action plan.

- **Check in on those around you.** Listen to what they are experiencing, and if they need assistance, see how you can help in a safe way.
- **Check in with yourself.** Be kind to yourself when things go wrong or if you didn't manage to get everything on your list done today. Make sure you're taking time to relax and unwind — and if you need help, please ask.
- **Choose kindness** towards ourselves and others. In our daily lives, we understand that kindness is the oil that greases the wheels and helps us to get through. In some places like New Zealand, even government bodies have adopted kindness as official advice: *Stay home, be kind.* Remember, this is a difficult time for everyone, and we never know what the other person may be experiencing, so when you can choose kind, take it.
- **Pause before reacting.** In uncertain times, it's easy to feel stressed, irritated and lash out at others, and that can make a tough situation worse. Try to pause and breathe before reacting, and consider whether you really need to make that comment. If you end up in an argument with people close to

you, try to address the rift as soon as possible, so that resentments don't fester.

- **Consider how you can help the most vulnerable.** In a crisis there is a risk that existing inequalities become entrenched and new ones emerge. Consider what you can do to help those in the community who may be vulnerable or struggling, or support agencies that do the work.
- **If you're in a leadership role,** pay attention to how you are communicating and make sure that you are listening and responding with empathy to the people you lead. People need to understand what is being asked of them, why it is being asked, and to have some recognition of the difficulties they are experiencing. (You can learn more about effective communication in chapter 7.)

Takeaway active listening tips

Active listening involves more than just hearing someone speak. When you practise active listening, you are fully concentrating on what is being said. You listen with all of your senses and give your full attention to the person speaking. Some features of active listening include:

- Being neutral and non judgemental
- Patience (periods of silence are not 'filled')
- Verbal and nonverbal feedback to show signs of listening (e.g. smiling, eye contact, leaning in, mirroring)
- Asking questions
- Reflecting back what is said
- Asking for clarification
- Summarising.

How to actively listen

Active listening is not something that just happens (that's hearing). It's an active process in which a conscious decision is made to listen to and understand the messages of the speaker — whether that's in the words they are saying, or something deeper.

You can try this exercise by yourself, or do it with someone else.

- Think of a time when you felt you weren't listened to (it could be at work, with family, at the doctor's, shopping, etc.)
- If you are doing this with a partner, share your stories. If you're doing this by yourself, try jotting down some notes in your journal.
- The listener must try to identify two things: what the person in the story did that demonstrated non-listening and what impact this had on the speaker. Hint: usually they feel devalued, angry, upset, or hurt.
- To debrief, gather all the ideas together and develop some principles of good listening by reversing what happened in the stories you were just thinking and talking about.

Next time you're listening to someone, think about how you can show you're really listening. Put that phone away, or at least have it face down if you need it with you.

Focus on listening to understand and empathise — not just to respond. Often we are just thinking about what we are going to say next rather than actually listening and understanding what the other person is saying. Take the time to truly listen, recognise emotion, and then respond to both the words and feelings that have been communicated.

Remember, there are cultural differences about how and when to maintain eye contact when listening, so make sure this doesn't result in misunderstandings about whether someone is actually listening or not.

Self-empathy

We've talked about showing empathy to others — but how about showing empathy to yourself?

We are living through times of unprecedented change. So much of what we took for granted about daily life in 2019 now feels out of reach. You may have kept yourself busy just trying to cope with the stresses and pressures of daily life, but that doesn't mean that all this change isn't taking a toll. This uncertainty is powerful enough to set even the least-anxious person on edge. Recognising that these are difficult times and consciously choosing to practise self-empathy will help you get through this time and stay well.

Self-empathy is not the same as self-compassion. Self-compassion involves treating yourself with the same kindness, concern and support you'd show to a good friend. Self-empathy means that one part of yourself 'observes', in an empathetic manner, another part of yourself that 'experiences'. This is done with an attitude of suspended judgement and openness towards yourself.

It sounds complex, but actually, self-empathy simply requires you to notice and recognise what is happening in you. We get in touch with our own sensations, emotions and thoughts. We feel into our body and observe our mind. We notice how our mind becomes distracted and how we start mind-wandering into memories or plans ahead. After a little while wandering, we pay attention to the distraction without judging and condemning it.

This is how the mind works; it focuses and then gets distracted for a while until we bring it back to focus. We learn to be aware of where our mind is and how our body feels moment to moment. In other words, we develop a mindful meta-awareness. And importantly, although we work to regulate our thoughts and our attention, we also accept ourselves as we are.

Self-empathy is also a stepping stone towards greater self-awareness. With self-empathy, we don't attempt to change the other person we are trying to help, as much as we transform ourselves in response to the other person. The recognition of an inner presence that can witness our own experience and recognise our own struggles, requires that we focus on ourselves rather than on the person we are trying to encourage, so that we can find an appropriate response.

It sounds counter-intuitive, and almost selfish, but self-empathy is actually a prerequisite for empathising with others. Self-empathy lies at the heart of how we can truly and effectively respond to others in times of distress and need. Unless you can notice what is going on for you in an empathetic way, it's very difficult for you to do that for others. It is only through self-empathy that we can accept others as they are and hold their pain lightly so that we can then offer meaningful support.

Feeling your feelings

One important part of practising self-empathy is learning to accept and feel your feelings. You may notice that you are feeling more tired than usual or more anxious than usual. You might find that some days you are optimistic and productive, while other days you struggle to focus. All of this is normal and likely to be exacerbated if you are facing renewed restrictions or lockdown.

You might also find yourself tempted to dismiss what you are feeling. Some say that we are the first generation to have feelings about our feelings. We minimise our pain and tell ourselves we should get over it, that we're not justified in feeling as we do, because others are suffering. We tell ourselves things like, '*I feel sad, but what have I really got to feel sad about? Other people have it worse.*' Yet we can be our own worst judges of what goes on in our heads and hearts.

We can — we should — stop at the first feeling. '*I feel sad. Let me spend five minutes feeling sad.*'

Your work is to feel your sadness, fear and anger, regardless of what someone else may or may not be feeling. Fighting your feelings doesn't help, because your body is still producing those feelings.

Self-empathy means that we can observe these feelings without condemnation and judgement, deal with them dispassionately or accept them as a part of what we are going through, rather than trying to deny them or squash them down. The more we struggle to understand that part of the human experience is experiencing a whole range of feelings, both pleasant and unpleasant, then the harder it is to get through life. That's not to say we just lie down and take whatever is coming, far from it. But it does mean recognising that we only have so much influence on issues outside of our control, and that also goes for our loved ones, neighbours, and work colleagues too.

Rather than entering into a struggle to quash these feelings, if we allow ourselves to experience them, for the vast majority of the time,[1] they peak and then pass on in a matter of moments, usually a few seconds, or a minute or two. We can move through them faster and feel empowered by, rather than be victims of, our feelings.

1. Verduyn, P & Lavrijsen, S (2015). Which emotions last longest and why: The role of event importance and rumination. *Motiv Emot*, 39:119–127.

CHAPTER 4

All the feels

We've seen how important it is to feel our feelings, and how accepting all our emotions helps us move through them quicker and be of real support to others. Now let's look at the kinds of emotions you might be experiencing during this pandemic and how you can process them.

One feeling I'd wager we have all experienced is worry. With so much change happening in every facet of life, it's normal to feel worried from time to time. We don't know how things are going to work out and that uncertainty creates a deep sense of discomfort.

Worry isn't a nice feeling or state of mind, yet we find ourselves going there over and over again. The hardest part of worrying about uncertain situations is the point where you start to spiral. In stressful times when we most need restorative rest, we can find ourselves lying awake in the wee small hours, worrying over things that we can't control. Your mind runs away with the worst-case scenario and you feel worse and worse.

If worry doesn't make us feel good, why do we do it? It seems to work like this. In the past, we've worried about something, but everything has turned out okay. The result is that our brain pairs the feeling of worry with a positive outcome. The brain becomes convinced that worrying helps us get the result that we want.

And sometimes it can. That dreadful feeling can motivate us into action and might help solve the problem. If we consider the fight or flight response, it seems likely that we evolved to experience worry in order to push us towards action when we need it.

But just like the fight or flight response, in our modern lives, worry often doesn't help at all and can actually make things harder. Severe worry is stressful. It prevents us from resting and relaxing. It hinders our ability to go about our day and take care of our lives. It takes control of our thoughts and saps our energy.

The good news is there are methods of dealing with these nagging feelings of dread and worry. We can't stop hurricanes, bad news, pandemics, or the clock; but it helps to acknowledge your worry and then focus on what you can control. Here's how.

1. Identify unproductive worrying

Productive worries tend to lead to actions that give us more control of our environment, whereas unproductive worries make us feel even more anxious and uncertain, and can become a vicious cycle. Try to differentiate how much of your worrying is productive (making sure there's enough food in the house) versus unproductive (staying up all night thinking about worst-case scenarios). If there's nothing you can do about it, it's not yours to worry over.

2. Express your worry

Instead of letting the worries go round and round in your head, try keeping a worry journal. Set aside a defined period of time — perhaps 15 minutes — when you will give yourself full permission to worry. Write all your fears and worries down in a notebook. Once the time is up, or you've run out of worries to record, put the notebook away and let it all go.

Your worry journal can act as a parking space for unproductive worries, so that they don't keep circling around your mind looking for a space to park. Many people find that by writing it all down they can interrupt the constant cycle of thoughts and move on, free to think about and do other things.

3. Practise mindfulness

Try to bring moments of mindfulness into your day, by sitting in active and intentional awareness. You can exercise mindfulness when sitting at the kitchen table eating your lunch: feel the chair under your body; appreciate the texture of the food as you chew; note the sensation of going from hungry to satisfied.

Mindfulness is not easy, but it's incredibly powerful. To hone the skill, you can practise mindfulness more formally through mindfulness meditation, which trains you to better manage racing thoughts and stay grounded and present when troubling uncertainty abounds.

4. Develop habits and routines for a sense of control

Much of the uncertainty comes from the lack of an end date to all the physical distancing, health threats, second or subsequent waves, and further lockdowns. When worry threatens to overwhelm you, it helps to recommit to your structure and routine, so you can feel a sense of control on a smaller, more individual scale. Choosing a few helpful habits, building them into your routines and sticking to them can help tame your worry more than you realise. Habits become automatic and give us a sense of predictability and control. Plus, when we complete a task, we feel a sense of accomplishment and that boosts our mood.

Habits and routines can help with any moment of uncertainty in life, well beyond this pandemic. Maybe you ended a relationship and feel aimless and confused about the future; or you moved across the country for a job to a town where you don't know a soul.

Not knowing how things will pan out is scary, but establishing some structure, building helpful habits into your routine and setting small, attainable goals can help you keep going. Try setting up an activity calendar (for work and fun stuff) and sticking to it as much as possible — even when you don't feel like it and would rather crash on the couch.

5. Seek out humour

Whether it's a TV show, funny tweets, or a group chat with friends, humour is very much about the here and now. The more we're in that headspace, the less our minds travel to the future and remind us of how uncertain it is.

6. Accept what you can't control

Acknowledging that we can't control and change everything is really important. This is easier said than done, but acceptance is a big step towards regaining peace of mind. Wanting to know and control everything fuels uncertainty, and obsessive consumption of information — grasping for certainty — can make things worse. Seeking out information is vital, and keeping up with news is important, but constantly refreshing your news and social media feeds only adds to your anxiety.

Find your circle of control

This exercise helps you to identify the things you can impact and the things that you can do nothing about, no matter how much you worry. This is an important step in being able to let some of that worry go.

1. Draw two circles — a circle of control and a circle of no influence.
2. Fill these two circles with all the things that you worry about.
3. Identify three positive actions you could take within your circle of control.

Did you find that much of what you worry about belongs in your circle of no influence? In uncertain times, it's most helpful if we focus on things that are within our control, like how we spend our time, making sure that we stay at home to protect ourselves and others, and checking in on loved ones to ensure they have what they need.

What your neighbour is doing is out of your influence or control. What is in your control is staying at least two metres from them, wearing a mask and washing your hands. Focus on that and let go of the neighbour's behaviour.

The same is true for national politics. You can't control what the politicians will do, but you can write to your representative and make your voice heard.

Doing something productive forces you to focus on that activity and interrupts the spiralling thoughts, easing some of that tension and anxiety. By choosing to do something useful that is within your circle of control, the feeling of worry begins to ease.

Grief

This may surprise you, but another emotion you may be feeling right now is grief — or even a number of different forms of grief. This is a normal emotion in the face of so much uncertainty.

The world has changed. We know this is temporary, but it doesn't feel that way, and in a sense, we also know that things will never return completely to the way they were. The loss of normalcy, the economic fallout and the loss of connection are painful. We are grieving all of these things collectively and that falls squarely outside our comfort zones.

As well as grieving for the things we have lost, we're also experiencing anticipatory grief. Anticipatory grief is that feeling we get when the future feels uncertain. We might feel anticipatory grief when we fear we might lose someone, like an ageing parent, or miss out on something we've looked forward to, like a wedding, graduation or travel plans. We can also feel anticipatory grief about things we hope for over the longer term, our imagined futures.

This kind of grief can feel very confusing. Our primal mind senses that there is a storm coming, or something bad is 'out there', but we can't see it. This breaks our sense of safety and we feel that loss not just individually or in our communities, but for people all around the globe. It's a strange feeling to us: a worldwide collective grief like we've never experienced in our lifetime.

So what can you do when you feel those waves of dread, loss or grief approaching?

A useful starting point is to understand the five stages of grief. This model was developed by psychologist Elisabeth Kübler-Ross in 1969, and defines the five most commonly observed states experienced by the grieving as denial, anger, bargaining, depression, and acceptance. It's interesting to observe how these stages have played out in our responses to Covid-19.

In the early days, we can see *denial*: This virus won't affect me/us.

There's *anger*: You're making me stay home and taking away my activities.

There's *bargaining*: Okay, if I physically distance for four weeks everything will be better, right?

There's *sadness*: I don't know when this will all end.

And, finally, there's *acceptance*: This is happening; I have to figure out how to proceed.

That's not to say we will progress neatly through these five stages to some conclusion. The model was never intended to be linear and no matter what sort of grief we are experiencing, it's common to jump back and forth between different stages, depending on what is happening at that time.

In the case of Covid-19, as we have seen resurgences of the virus around the world, we've also seen corresponding rising tides of anger, denial, bargaining, sadness and sometimes acceptance, as each new encounter with the pandemic produces different measures that we need to adapt to. The grief persists because the counter-factual remains the same: if we don't take action, we will still have grief, but most likely at a far greater scale, with loss of lives, economic livelihoods, and, very possibly, entire communities.

Though we may find ourselves experiencing different stages of grief at different times, this final stage of acceptance is perhaps where the power resides, because that is where we can find things that we can control. *I can wash my hands. I can keep a safe distance. I can wear a mask. I can learn how to work virtually.*

With anticipatory grief, it might feel harder to find things you can control and take positive action, because your mind goes to the future and begins to anticipate the worst-case scenarios. Your mind tries to protect you and activate your threat alert system by showing you grim images. This is where unhealthy anticipatory grief becomes anxiety.

When that happens, your goal is not to ignore those images or to try to make them go away — your mind won't let you do that and it can be painful to try to force it. The goal is to find balance in the things you're thinking. If you feel the worst image taking shape, make yourself think of the best image. *We all get a little sick and the world continues. Not everyone I love dies. Maybe no one I love dies because we're all taking the right steps.* Neither scenario should be ignored, but neither should be allowed to dominate.

To calm yourself, bring yourself into the present with a mindfulness practice. It can be as simple as naming five things in the room. There's a couch, a chair, a picture of your family, an old blanket, and a TV. Breathe. Realise that in the present moment, nothing you've anticipated or worried about has happened. In this moment, you're okay. You have food. You are not sick. Tune into your senses and think about what they are telling you. The couch is comfortable. The blanket smells of your dog (in a good way). I can hear the birds outside the window.

People are often surprised at how useful this simple exercise can be. It really does help to move you through the immediate pain you may experience.

If you still feel overwhelmed with grief from time to time, be assured that you are not alone. Language gives us the power to be able to name our internal experiences and there is something powerful about naming what we are feeling as grief. It helps us truly feel what's inside of us, and to come to a better understanding and perhaps not feel so alone.

When you name your emotion, you can feel it and let it move through you. In one study,[1] it was confirmed that sadness was found to be the longest-lasting emotion whereas shame, surprise, fear, disgust, being touched, irritation, and relief were the shortest. But even sadness passed too. So, give yourself permission to stop and experience the grief. Let it move through you. And then let's keep going.

Grief and the loss of a loved one

Sadly, many people have experienced especially cruel losses and disappointments during this pandemic, like losing a loved one, or being unable to say goodbye and knowing that your loved one died alone. This form of grief has emerged as one of the most challenging aspects of living through this time.

Although many societies around the world have become perhaps less formally religious in recent decades, we still maintain traditions and rituals around death, and many of these are deeply culturally ingrained and meaningful.

The physical distancing protocols that have been necessary to control the spread of the coronavirus means that many have had

1. Verduyn, P & Lavrijsen, S (2015). Which emotions last longest and why: The role of event importance and rumination. *Motiv Emot*, 39:119–127.

to bear their grief and loss in solitude, without the opportunity to come together to join in ritual and mourning, and without social support from close friends and family. Antonio Cana, a doctor in an overwhelmed hospital in Madrid said, 'That's the cruellest thing about this pandemic. The thousands who have died from Covid-19, passing away alone. In a hospital ward or a room in an old people's home. Without family members near them. Not one goodbye or farewell.'[2]

The Covid-19 pandemic has led to delayed grieving processes for many, and not only those who have lost loved ones to the virus. Many have found themselves unable to attend funerals, or have travelled across borders to say final farewells, only to find themselves trapped in quarantine, having to say their last goodbyes over Skype. The moment of saying goodbye to a family member is a critical part of the process of mourning. The reality that this is not possible has been reported to bring new and different kinds of sadness, affecting both individuals and whole families and communities.

We know that a deficit in social support for those in a mourning process may cause the progression through the grieving process to be more drawn out, or negatively impact the health of those in mourning. It is difficult to distinguish between the sense of loneliness and isolation caused by this complicated grieving process and the physical isolation that may have been imposed by regulations. It has all got so horribly complex and sad.

Óscar Fernández and Miguel González-González have written[3]

2. Fernández, Ó & González-González, M (2020). The Dead with No Wake, Grieving with No Closure: Illness and Death in the Days of Coronavirus in Spain. *J Relig Health*.
3. Fernández, Ó & González-González, M (2020). The Dead with No Wake, Grieving

about how grieving has become another dimension of community life to be re-invented in the present social context. They underline how important it is that we do not take physical distancing to mean social distancing, and that this is especially true when thinking about those trying to find closure for their sadness in the face of the death of a loved one who has not been viewed, waked, or farewelled.

In other words, if you experienced the loss of a loved one during this time, it's important that you allow yourself time and space to grieve, and seek help if you need it. If a friend is in that situation, reach out and offer support however you can. Depending on your current restrictions, you may not be able to give or receive a hug, but there are many ways to show someone that they are not alone.

Putting on a brave face

In times of uncertainty, many people feel like they need to put on a brave face, for their children or for others that care about them, even though they may be feeling very differently on the inside. Should you ever just pretend to be happy when you're not? The answer is more complex than you might think.

Faking happiness doesn't count as happiness, of course; it won't bring all the positive benefits that real happiness will. But when you paste on a smile there *is* something at work that is pretty amazing: facial expressions themselves can actually make us feel. If you wrinkle your nose and narrow your eyes as you would if you were really angry, your body will release some adrenaline and your heart rate may speed up as if you were actually angry.

with No Closure: Illness and Death in the Days of Coronavirus in Spain. *J Relig Health.*

The same thing is true for other emotions. This means that sometimes we should just smile, even if we don't feel like it. As horribly forced as that sounds, there is solid science to back up the notion that this will, in fact, make us feel happier.

Facial expression alone, without even feeling the corresponding emotion, is enough to create noticeable changes in your autonomic nervous system. Force a smile and crinkle your eyes, and your body will release all kinds of feel-good brain chemicals into your system.

You can even try holding a pencil between your teeth — which activates your smile muscles — and you will likely find that your heart rate goes down and you start to feel calmer, happier. One study shows that you'll also find things funnier for a while (but you may also start to drool).

I'm not advocating that we force ourselves or our children to smile when we're in the thick of bad feelings. When kids are feeling anxious or just pretty rubbish, we need to emotion-coach them so that they learn to deal with their negative emotions. This means helping them to name the emotions, find ways to express that feeling in a safe way, and learn skills to help them to move on and become absorbed in activity that will helpfully move them on to another range of experiences.

If you've dealt with your negative emotions and are ready to feel better, by all means paste on that smile if that's what you need to do.

Just remember to create some space for you to be with your vulnerabilities in a safe way. For you, that might be reaching out to family and friends — or it might be talking to someone who isn't immediately connected with you if that feels safer right now. That might mean reaching out to a mental health service or a counselling helpline in your area.

So, yes — sometimes it's necessary to put on a brave face. I get it. Just don't forget that even superheroes change out of their costumes and let the mask slip when in the company of their trusted besties. Take the time to do that for yourself too.

Prioritise the Fabulous Four

If all this feels like doom and gloom, then it's time to bring a little joy back.

One way to be kind and empathetic to yourself is by consciously prioritising activities that make you feel good. When you're feeling low you tend to be less active than normal and you might stop doing things that lift your spirits. You can end up just blobbing and this can make you feel even worse. This is also known as the exhaustion funnel. This concept from Dr Marie Åsberg from the Karolinska Institute summarises a downward spiral of unhappiness, anxiety and even more stress. In the book *Mindfulness: A Practical Guide to Finding Peace in a Frantic World*,[4] Professor Mark Williams and Dr Danny Penman discuss the idea of this further: As you get busier, you start giving up something in your life to make room for 'important' stuff, like work and being busy. What usually happens is you decide to give up your rewarding and nourishing things like family time and recreation and you start to think of them as 'optional'. All the things you enjoy, they can wait. You tell yourself that you're just putting them on the back burner for a little while and you'll get back to them soon. You are then left with nothing but work and other daily stresses in your life that drain you like an energy vampire. You end up totally depleted and exhausted.

4. Williams, M & Penman, D (2011). *Mindfulness: A Practical Guide to Finding Peace in a Frantic World*. Little, Brown.

To pull yourself out of the funnel, it can help hugely to do activities from which you derive pleasure or feel a sense of achievement. Sometimes we don't value ourselves highly enough to allow ourselves to experience pleasure. We put other people's needs first, and send ourselves to the back of the queue, seeing pleasure as something to enjoy 'when we get around to it'. But life is busy, so the danger is that we never get around to it. This is especially true for some parents, who put their children's needs so much above their own that they give themselves no personal time and space at all.

Even if you don't think you *deserve* to enjoy yourself right now (and truly: you do), bringing pleasure into life is a fundamental plank of personal resilience. Pleasurable activities like engaging in the hobbies and interests that you've let slip over the last while, or doing the things you enjoyed when you were younger before life got so much more complex, can help enormously to ease depressive feelings. The same goes for exercise, social connection and activities that bring a sense of achievement, like reaching small goals, or purposeful work.

Part of the issue here is that we tend to neglect the things that nourish us in favour of just getting through — and that makes uncertainty so much harder to bear. That's why it's important that whatever structure you create for your week includes a good mix of the 'Fabulous Four': pleasurable, physical, social and achievement activities.

When you have a good mix of all four, you can arrest any further fall into the exhaustion funnel. Not only that, but your Fab Four will help you to build a ladder to a place where interesting and pleasurable activities are a regular part of your weekly schedule again, instead of the first thing that gets cancelled when other tasks or obligations disrupt your week.

Incorporating the Fab Four

Step 1 Identify activities you could do which fit into each of the following categories:

- Pleasurable activities
- Achievement-based activities
- Physical activities
- Social activities.

Step 2 Make a balanced schedule across your week.

It's important to do a balance of activities from each group. So, for example, each day try scheduling in an activity from a different group to the day before. Of course, some activities might fit into more than one group — a virtual or in-person coffee and cake with friends can be both pleasurable and sociable.

Making a conscious effort to bring the Fab Four into your week will go a long way to lift your spirits and find joy in life, even during tough times. The Fab Four also provides an alternative framework for fulfilling some of your Five Ways to Wellbeing (connect, give, notice, learn, stay active) from chapter 2.

Keep a journal

Many people find that keeping a private journal (as distinct from public, online blogging or posting) provides a safe space for them to reveal their innermost feelings. There is evidence that once we have written our feelings down on paper, we can start to feel less troubled by difficult emotions, and they're less likely to go round and round our bodies and minds, crowding out any space for other, more uplifting emotions.

Now when you think about journaling, you might have an image of a pretty notebook in the hands of a teenage girl trying to find herself and dealing with teen drama. In fact, many of the world's top leaders and influencers from the past to the modern day, from Marcus Aurelius to Marie Curie, from Lady Gaga to Tim Ferriss, kept or keep a journal.

Journaling can be a really powerful way of helping you stay on top of things during difficult experiences. Keeping a journal can make us more aware (and self-aware!), helping us detect sneaky, unhealthy patterns in our thoughts and behaviours. That allows us to take more control over our lives and puts things in perspective. It can also help us shift from a negative mindset to a more positive one, especially about ourselves.

Effective journaling requires more than a 'brain dump' onto the page. To get the full benefits, write in a private and personalised space that is free from distractions. Keep your journal private and for your eyes only — not your spouse, not your family, not your friends. Aim to write at least once each day, and during intense or particularly stressful times, try to write at least three or four times in a day if you can. If you're on the go, you can just jot out some thoughts on your phone and transfer it to your journal later.

Wondering what to write about? Well, WRITE turns out to be a useful acronym.

W — What topic? What do you want to write about? What's going on for you? How do you feel? What are you thinking about? What do you want? Name it.

R — Review or reflect on your topic. Close your eyes. Take three deep breaths. Focus. You can start with 'I feel ...' or 'I want ...' or 'I think ...' or 'Today, ...' or 'Right now, ...' or 'In this moment, ...'

I — Investigate your thoughts and feelings. Start writing and keep writing. Follow the pen or your fingers on the keyboard. If you get stuck or run out of juice, close your eyes and re-centre yourself. Reread what you've already written and continue writing.

T — Time yourself. Write for 5–15 minutes. Write the start time and the projected end time at the top of the page. Use the timer on your watch, cellphone or oven.

E — Exit well, by rereading what you've written and reflecting on it in a sentence or two: 'As I read this, I notice ...' or 'I'm aware of ...' or 'I feel ...'. Note any action steps to take.

Your journal will not only help you process what's happening for you, but in years to come it will be a fascinating record of this incredible time in history.

Our emotional lives are such an important part of how we get through a crisis. That includes developing an awareness of how the crisis affects those we care about and, most importantly, how it impacts upon us and influences our decisions.

Self-awareness, a focus on others, acceptance, and action: these pillars of empathy can help us all get through tough times in better shape. And it starts with us.

By practising self-empathy through carefully observing our own experience without judgement and by learning to cope with our own difficult emotions, we then start to be able to be more open to understanding the experience of others. That puts us in a better place to make good decisions about how to help ourselves and each other.

CHAPTER 5

Staying connected

Decades of research overwhelmingly shows that the number one factor that helps us adapt to challenging circumstances is social support.[1] The more connected and supported we feel, the better we are able to adapt to and handle what is right in front of us.

We feel supported when we are cared for, when we know that help is available from others if we need it and when we are part of a supportive social network. That support can come in many forms, from emotional support to the provision of information advice, practical support like financial assistance or help getting jobs done, and social support, or a sense of companionship and belonging.

And it's not just actual support that counts. Even the perception that support is available should we need it can be enough to help lower our stress levels and ease mental distress, particularly if that support is from family and friends. Support from communities and agencies is also important because they form a wider part of the ecosystem from which we draw support. Although we might like to think of ourselves as autonomous individuals, we rely on others for support. We are built that way, whether we are consciously aware of it or not.

Taking time to build up supportive relationships is one of the best things you can do to support your mental wellbeing in uncertain

---

1. Ministry of Health (2016). *Framework for Psychosocial Support in Emergencies.* Wellington: Ministry of Health.

times, or build your resilience in case of the inevitable future life challenges you will encounter. Having someone to confide in, be it a relative, partner or a friend, is one of the most important forms of protection from becoming depressed when something bad happens. If you don't have a close supportive relationship, or if your friends do not provide you with the support you need, then it's worth making the effort to build up this support.

Building supportive relationships takes time and effort. As an immigrant to New Zealand from the other side of the planet, I know this only too well. It doesn't happen overnight. When building relationships seems difficult, it is helpful to remember that it can be done at any stage of life and that there are many steps along the way.

1. **Meet new people.** Put yourself in people's way by making contact with groups of people with similar interests, neighbours, clubs, voluntary groups.
2. **Build a friendship.** Focus on shared experiences, activities and pleasures. Do things together. Don't wait to be invited, be the one who suggests an activity and try to keep a lightness about their response to your invitation. If they say no, try not to take rejection personally. If the other person is also feeling isolated, they might find it hard to commit to someone or something new. Ask again another time, or ask someone else.
3. **Consolidate friendships.** Keep in touch. Make regular contact. Become a good listener as well as a good talker. Try to keep in contact even when you are not feeling social or embarrassed about imposing on someone.
4. **Nurture your friendships.** Look for ways to show you care, in good times as well as bad. Tolerate people's moments of bad temper, grumpiness or silence.
5. **Use your friendships for mutual support.** Don't run away from people when you are feeling low. And don't turn away

from friends when they need someone to turn to. Try to offer a listening, empathetic ear — and remember, empathy works best with an action plan. Note, though, that a supportive relationship must not be a smothering one — we need our own independence and autonomy as well as support.

Of course, even if you have strong connections, all of these restrictions and lockdowns mean it hasn't always been possible to connect with people as we might like. So how can you cultivate your social wellbeing in the middle of a pandemic while doing all the right things like staying at home to protect you, your loved ones, and the wider community from infection?

When the pandemic began unfolding rapidly in March 2020, I asked my parents in the UK to go into voluntary isolation to keep themselves safe. Since then, we have had several heart-wrenching and difficult conversations about what this would mean for them, their ability to see family — and especially grandchildren — both close to them in London and here in New Zealand. There were no easy answers, but we made a commitment to keep talking to each other on a daily basis, and keep our connections going no matter how difficult things might get.

The obvious solution is technology. People often blame technology as a cause of loneliness, pointing out that we spend too much time scrolling through social media and not enough of it interacting in real life. But recent research paints a more nuanced picture: *how* you use such platforms seems to matter more than *how much* you do so. We can all benefit from developing digital habits that support meaningful human connections — especially now that it may be an ongoing option until we get on top of the pandemic.

Here are a few suggestions for how to connect without physical contact, by using technology in socially healthy ways.

1. Face to face from afar. The next best thing to in-person interaction is video chat, because facial cues, body language and other nonverbal forms of communication are important for bonding. When possible, opt for video over messaging or calling, and play around with doing what you would normally do with others. For example, try having a digital dinner with someone new you meet on a dating app, a virtual coffee meeting with friends or a remote book club meeting.

2. Practise one-minute kindness. Getting lots of likes on a social media post may give you a fleeting hit of dopamine, but receiving a direct message or email with a genuine compliment or expression of gratitude is more personal and longer lasting — without taking much more time. When you find yourself scrolling through people's posts, stop and send one of them a few kind words. After all, we need a little extra kindness to counter the stress and uncertainty of this coronavirus.

3. Deepen or broaden your connections. Fundamentally, there are two ways to overcome loneliness: nurture your existing relationships or form new ones. Reflect on your current state of social health and then take one digital action to deepen it — such as getting in touch with a friend or family member you haven't spoken with in a while — or one digital action to broaden it — such as reaching out to someone you'd like to get to know.

4. Use a conversation prompt. Increasingly, apps and social platforms are being designed to help us optimise our online interactions with loved ones. But also consider using conversation prompts, such as TableTopics or The And (www.theand.us), to spark interesting conversation during a video call — just to mix things up a little.

5. Frequency beats duration. Okay, this is not always true, but it often helps to have quick, frequent check-ins, rather than less-frequent, longer conversations. My parents live half a world away, but I don't call them once a week for a long catch-up; I call them every day for a short time. That works for me and them — figure out what works for you and your loved ones.

6. It's okay to be boring. We may not have much to report to each other but social connection is valuable even if there's not much to say. Set up that Zoom call to create an atmosphere of being together in parallel, even if you don't want to 'say' anything.

Group calls can also be useful for older kids who are homeschooling, to re-create the sense of being in a classroom or library. On a group call, they all do their work or thing silently (they put themselves on mute so they don't hear the sounds of each other typing, etc.), but they can see each other, so they feel together and they can unmute themselves if they have something to say.

Loneliness

What if you do all that and still feel lonely? In many places in the world, loneliness is already something many people struggle with on a daily basis. When social distancing and lockdowns were first imposed, many experts raised concerns that loneliness would get worse.

Interestingly, some studies carried out in the US over the initial phases of social distancing and movement restrictions suggest that didn't happen. While loneliness did increase a bit, the rise was nowhere near as steep or significant as expected.

So why didn't people report dramatically more loneliness at a time when most were more physically distant from other people and normal routines were disrupted more than ever before? We don't really know, but researchers have put forward some ideas.

The sense of solidarity that people feel when they are collectively under some threat or going through a challenge together is thought to be a strong protective factor, and certainly proved stronger than researchers anticipated at the outset. While a sense of coming together has been recognised as protective in other disaster situations, what's interesting here is that sense of solidarity seemed to hold up even when people could not physically come together. As the pandemic public health measures forced many stores and businesses to close temporarily, neighbours began to rely on each other more. However, as repeated lockdowns and other restrictions take place over time, this sense of solidarity might start to erode — and, indeed, there are worrying signs that this has happened already.

Another possible reason is that social pressure to participate in activities was released — this idea of fear of missing out, or FOMO, where we track who's going out to the party, or who's going out to events, and perhaps feel left out or rejected. When everyone is staying home, this is far less of an issue.

People could also connect with each other in non-physical ways, like online catch-ups with family and friends, hunting teddy bears, or neighbourhood front-doorstep workouts. These were healthy ways to keep connected during a crisis.

For now, we may have avoided a great flood of loneliness, but that's not to say it won't yet unfold over time or with the resurgence of the virus in current or future waves.

If you do find yourself feeling lonely or isolated, there's one simple thing you can do to help yourself feel a little love and care no matter what your situation: discover the magic of touch.

Humans are wired to be touched. From birth until the day we die, our need for physical contact is constant. Being touch starved —

also known as skin hunger or touch deprivation — occurs when a person experiences little to no touch from other living things. If you live alone, that can be really, really hard especially in lockdown, and even more so if you don't have a pet to keep you company that you can stroke or touch (because pets can really help).

One of the brain chemicals underlying the positive effects of touch is oxytocin. Oxytocin is responsible for parent-infant bonding as well as many other situations that are related to human bonding and wellbeing.

The release of oxytocin normally occurs in response to closeness in good relationships; but the interesting thing is that the wellbeing effects can be mimicked to a certain extent by massage and stroking of the skin. And the really interesting thing is that you can also get some of these effects without another person. Stroking your own skin, or even just gently pressing on your own skin, can mimic the effects enough that you can start the release of oxytocin in your body, which helps to lift your mood and make you feel better.

Practising self-compassion in this way is actually really simple. One easy way to soothe and comfort yourself when you're feeling bad is to give yourself a gentle hug or caress, or simply put your hand on your heart and feel the warmth of your hand. It may feel awkward or embarrassing at first, but your body doesn't know that. It just responds to the physical gesture of warmth and care, just as a baby responds to being cuddled in its mother's arms.

Our skin is an incredibly sensitive organ and research indicates that physical touch releases oxytocin, provides a sense of security, soothes distressing emotions, and calms cardiovascular stress. So why not try it?

If you notice that you're feeling tense, upset, sad or self-critical, or

lonely, try stroking your arm or face, or gently rocking your body. What's important is that you make a clear gesture that conveys feelings of love, care and tenderness. If other people are around, you can often fold your arms in a non-obvious way, gently squeezing yourself in a comforting manner. You can also simply imagine hugging or caressing yourself if you can't make the actual physical gesture.

Try stroking your skin or putting your hand over your heart during difficult periods several times a day for a period of at least a week. Give it a try —you've got nothing to lose.

Relationships with a significant other

So what about intimate relationships? How do emergencies impact on the relationship you may have with a significant other?

While a crisis can highlight the strengths of intimate relationships, it can expose the problems too.

In 'normal' times, most couples spend a large part of an average day apart, since one partner or both work outside of the home. Since Covid-19 hit, many couples have been required to spend all day at home together, either through lockdown or extended periods of working from home. As well as spending 24/7 together, circumstances threw in some other common stressors, like dramatic changes in routine, anxiety about health, potential unemployment, financial insecurity, juggling caregiving or homeschooling for children, worries about elderly relatives, lack of social connection outside of the home and general uncertainty about the future.

Being around each other's idiosyncrasies all day (and night), while trying to cope with these stressors, can bring up issues that had

been bubbling under the surface. Any vulnerabilities will be brought into the light.

In addition, couples may use different coping mechanisms to deal with stress. For instance, one spouse may be preoccupied with risk; the other may be focused on keeping life as regular as possible. One spouse might take a proactive approach; the other may be more passive and hopeless. These differences make couples clash and this polarisation can end the relationship, if the couple doesn't take steps to do something about it.

We know that applications for divorce increased in some Chinese cities as they emerged from lockdown. We also know that domestic violence can increase in times of isolation. If you witness or are involved in an emergency situation where someone is being hurt or threatened with violence, call the police immediately. You might save someone from being injured or killed. In an emergency situation, you do not need permission from the person being hurt to ring police.

If it is not an emergency situation, but you know someone is being abused by a partner, ex-partner or family member, the best thing to do is to build trust with that person, and offer non judgemental support and information about specialist domestic violence services. Make sure they know that you won't share anything they tell you about their situation unless they want you to, or unless it is an emergency situation and they are being hurt — or are at risk of being hurt — at that moment.

Take their lead and find out what is important to them. They know their partner (or whoever is controlling/abusing them) better than anyone, and will already be trying and doing things (often restricting their own freedom) to keep themselves — and their children — safe. Think about how you can support their efforts or make more choices available to them.

So what can you do to help your relationship survive through stressful times? Here are a few tips that will help you and your significant other hold on to each other and your relationship.

Pick and choose your battles. Make sure you don't react to everything your partner does that annoys you. If your partner is moody, remember it's probably not really about you. Give them extra slack. Within reason.

Do not harp on about relationship problems. Put a limit (e.g. 20 minutes, once a day) on discussing difficult issues. And when it's over, put it aside. Perhaps, plan a 'conflict/concern time' in your schedule. Also, have a rule that either of you can call a timeout if it gets too heated and you will resume the discussion later.

Carve out alone time. If you have the luxury of multiple rooms, create some time for yourself in a different room. If you don't have a separate room, use headphones to create artificial boundaries.

Be engaged socially with other people. For example, if you're isolating or confined to your home, schedule wine and dine with your friends and family through FaceTime or Zoom or host a game night by playing virtual games. That way your partner is not the only adult you interact with and you'll both feel the joy of connecting with friends.

Don't get ahead of yourself with financial matters. Try to focus your attention on ways to survive throughout the remainder of the crisis. Try not to look too far ahead, as the future is unpredictable. During a crisis, try sticking to taking each day and week as it comes.

Choose intimacy. A common remedy for conflict — and a way to increase closeness — is sex. This might not be top of mind while you are worried about infection, finances and the kids. But romantic connection is even more useful than ever. However, if your partner is not up for sex, don't nag or shame, and definitely don't coerce, because that will make them feel worse. Hand holding, hugging, offering a massage, or anything soothing and comforting can be connecting in and of itself.

Get help. If you and your partner need more help, seek relationship counselling. Having a therapist to talk to about some of the challenges arising can be really helpful. Many counsellors and therapists now offer individual or couple sessions over Zoom, so you won't even have to leave the house.

The magic five

No matter how strong your relationship, it's important to realise that some kind of conflict is pretty much inevitable in stressful times. The difference between happy and unhappy couples is the balance between positive and negative interactions during arguments.

To have a happy relationship you need to counteract every negative interaction you have in an argument with five positive interactions.[2]

So what are the negative interactions we need to watch out for? You'd think anger would be one of them, right? Yes, but there is an 'and' to that. Anger can certainly be part of a negative interaction, but it's most damaging when it's paired with criticism or contempt, or if it is defensive anger.

Being emotionally dismissive is another no-no. Couples need to be

2. A good place to start reading more about this: Gottman, JM & Schwartz-Gottman (2017). The Natural Principles of Love. *Journal of Family Theory & Review*, 9:7–26.

aware of subtle negatives such as facial expressions. Four negative qualities are the strongest predictors for divorce: contempt, criticism, defensiveness, and stonewalling. Eye-rolling has emotional power as it seems to be interpreted as a signal of one or more of these negative qualities; research shows eye-rolling after a spouse's comment can be a strong predictor for divorce.

Eye-rolling suggests contempt. Empathy and contempt are polar opposites. Empathy involves caring about others' feelings and concerns. Contempt is arrogant disregard, dismissal, and denigration of others' concerns ('I know best'). Empathy nurtures relationship bonds; contempt invites problems.

It's not likely that stopping the eye-rolling will save your marriage, but it's a good indicator that something is going on that needs to be addressed.

These negative interactions have a great deal of emotional power, which is why it takes five positive interactions to overcome any negative interactions. While negative interactions appear in healthy relationships too, they're quickly repaired with validation and empathy. Arguments in these relationships tend also to start more gently, and couples tend to make minor repairs as soon as they hit bumps in the road.

Here are some positive interactions that appear in flourishing relationships:

1. Be interested. When your partner raises something, do you listen? Do you show how closely you're listening by asking questions — and by paying attention to how you ask them?

2. Show affection. Do you hold hands with your partner? Do you embrace them at the end of the day? Displays of affection — and they don't have to be public — can happen in small ways both inside and outside of any conflict that might be happening in your relationship.

3. Small gestures add up. Demonstrating in small ways that your partner matters and doing this often creates a buffer of positivity in your relationship. This helps you to engage in more positive interactions when the relationship temporarily rubs against the rails.

4. Find opportunities for agreement. An alliance in an argument — an area you can agree upon, however minor — can fundamentally change how you argue. By agreeing even a little, you're showing that you can see your partner's point of view as valid and that you care about them.

5. Empathise and apologise. If your partner is upset with something you said or did, and if you can find a moment in the argument, simply apologise. *I'm sorry I hurt your feelings and did that. It makes me sad that I hurt you.* This simple apology provides positive and empathetic fuel that actually helps to strengthen your bond.

6. Accept your partner's perspective even if you disagree with it. Validation of your partner's perspective doesn't mean that you agree with them, but it does show you respect them.

7. Make jokes. If you've got inside or private jokes that only each other would understand, this highlights your exclusivity and your bond with each other. Take care though — playful, silly jokes have their place in defusing an argument, but belittling and laughing 'at' your partner does not.

Share this list with your partner and make a commitment to fostering positive interactions every day. You might even want to copy this list out and stick it on the fridge as a daily reminder to cherish the love you have and protect your relationship.

CHAPTER 6

Supporting kids through Covid-19

Covid-19 has been tough on kids. Even if relatively few have experienced serious illness, they've missed out on school, time with friends and extended family, and important rites of passage. For teens there's the added challenge of all the developmental and hormonal changes going on, while our young adults — Generation Z — are beginning their adult lives in a world of uncertainty.

Just as adults are struggling with uncertainty, so are our kids. They might have faced disruption to their schooling with no understanding of when things turn to normal. They might be missing seeing friends or extended family in real life. And some will experience fear and anxiety about what happens next, not only for themselves but for family members who may be far away.

Children react differently to stress compared with adults. They may become withdrawn, or act in a more 'babyish' or younger-than-their-years way. They may seem anxious or clingy, or be preoccupied with illness in their play or drawing. Stress might show itself through sleeping issues or nightmares, or getting physical symptoms like stomach aches or headaches. If these become persistent, then it might be time to get some help.

Some kids will incorporate the coronavirus into their play, as a way to express what's going on for them in manageable ways. Just as children experiencing wartime may enact battle or fight scenes in their play, kids might dress up like superheroes and pretend to go out and save the world by killing the coronavirus, plan their end-of-lockdown party, play Covid-tag, pretend to be sick, or tell someone else to pretend to cough or be short of breath.

While it may feel unsettling to play 'illness', this sort of pretend play is a healthy and normal way for children to process stressful emotions and experiences. Pretend play is often a sign that a child is working through something they are finding pretty intense — like living through a global pandemic — and processing how that is showing up in their lives.

Play actually helps children to regulate their mood when perhaps they're finding their experiences overwhelming. Through pretend play and role-playing, they can get some distance, and experience it less intensely. This also helps them to be able to integrate the experience, including their fears of what is happening and what might happen in the future. They can then build a story around it.

The narrative they construct around the play is the important part. What happens in the story matters far more than the appearance of coronavirus in their play. Studies have shown that children who incorporate their experience of being in hospital into their play, by performing surgeries on their teddy bears, for example, experience less anxiety than those who don't play like this.

Children's play tends to reflect what they are experiencing in the world around them, what they see in the media, and what they hear from conversations among adults. That's why we need to be mindful about the media that children get exposed to and what they hear in our conversations, and remember, kids have got bat ears — they pick up everything.

Play can also help a child regain a sense of control. If a child is creating a box and putting dolls and stuffed toys inside and asking them to stay inside, then this might be reflecting their understanding of quarantine or isolation. But they're the one giving the commands and making the requests, meaning they, in a sense, are taking some control of the situation.

So if your child needs to put on a cape and turn the virus into a bad guy in their superhero make-believe, then that might bring them a sense of relief from anxiety. The coronavirus is the new bogey man, the scary monster that lives under the bed, or in the cupboard in the back of the room whose door should never, ever be left open at night. For children, pretend play is a very powerful way of working through all that's happening right now.

The main thing to watch out for is repeated play where things don't seem to move on, or don't get resolved. If you get repeated play with no resolution, then that's where you might need to get more involved. If children becoming clingy or upset during play, and this doesn't seem to be changing, that's another sign that you might want to help that play along, or get some help with doing that.

You can learn more about your child's understanding of what's going on in their world by following their lead in their play. By listening to them tell the story, you'll gain an insight into how your child is making meaning of these events and expose any gaps in understanding they may have.

For younger kids, you can help them build that meaning and understanding through play. You could have them practise physical distancing through their dolls or stuffed toys. You can count the number of ways they can greet each other without touching each other. Or perhaps they want to play doctor or patient.

Don't stop them from trying to figure stuff out on their own, and try not to guide their play too much, but give them answers or set up simple options. Make a note of anything that is incorrect, plan a way to give them correct information later and see how it shows up in their play another time further along the track.

If older children are playing Covid-tag, don't just tell them to stop. Take a moment to explain why that might be scary and ask why they were using the virus as the thing to run away from.

Finally, this might be the perfect time to let go and get into that pretend play! If your child says 'You be this and I'll be that', follow your child's lead — you might enjoy it. It will help you escape from reality for a minute, it will show your child that you are there for them, and it will help them work out their emotions and fears as they see you reacting in this safe, contained, pretend space.

So if they want to play coronavirus, let them. Guide them through understanding and by answering questions, but don't stop them from trying to figure it out for themselves through play.

Homeschooling

One of the more difficult and unexpected challenges of parenting through this pandemic has been homeschooling. For many families, homeschooling was not something they had considered undertaking before and certainly not in circumstances where everyone was forced to stay at home all the time.

But with school closures and lockdowns, parents had no choice but to pick up the education load; no easy task at the best of times, let alone while juggling other responsibilities and worries, working from home, trying to keep a business afloat or perhaps leaving the house to work as essential workers.

As we move in and out of restrictions, many of us are realising we may have to take on additional periods of homeschooling now or in the future. Make no mistake about it; homeschooling in a pandemic is not a 'normal' experience. This is not teaching as we know it so it's important to go easy on yourself — and your kids — as you adapt.

No matter what your child's age, educators recommend providing structure if they're staying home from school and by now you know this must be balanced with liberal doses of empathy too. Structure and empathy are key to getting through a stressful time — and homeschooling is no exception to this.

The big picture here is that this balance of structure and empathy helps your child to become more self-regulated. This skill of being able to manage their activity and their emotions will continue to be beneficial for them long after this pandemic is over. In fact, it's likely that kids with good emotional self-regulation skills will cope better with everything that is going on. These are skills that can be learned and refined as kids go through different experiences. This pandemic is one of those experiences, so explaining the current crisis, how it's unfolding and enlisting your child's help in making the best of a bad situation is important.

Remember, your child will be missing their usual routine; where they go, who they spend time with, their usual way of doing things. Remember to understand all this is difficult for them too. It's likely you'll see signs of frustration. Remember to listen to their concerns and be flexible about the structure you set up. It most likely won't work every day, but it gives you something to work with and adapt.

As a parent, that goes for you too. Do your best, and at times, just do what you need to to get by safely and healthily. Social media can be a curse at times like this when we can feel like everyone else is doing a better job than we are. Remember that social media is a cultivated showcase that people want you to see. They're not showing you the messy office, the sink full of dirty dishes, or the hour they spent trying to referee continually bickering kids.

Recognise there will be both good and bad days, and everything in between, and that this is just how it is right now.

Here are some tips to make homeschooling work for your family:

- **Make a plan.** Work with teachers and other parents to get a sense of what is going to work in your family. What are the 'must-haves'? What are the 'nice-to-haves'? Do you have to do two Zoom meetings a day, or is it enough for the kids to show up once? What can you do on those days when you feel like you can barely get yourself together to speak a full sentence, let alone impart any kind of wisdom or stick to any curriculum? Get clear on the teacher's expectations and be clear about your own constraints in return.
- **Set up a designated schoolwork space.** When home becomes the space for everything, it's good to have a designated space for schoolwork. Not everyone's personal circumstances are going to allow for this, but if you can at least have a space away from toys, gadgets, phones and tablets, it gives your child a better chance of staying on task. And if that is not possible, then perhaps the space becomes a schoolwork-only zone during designated time periods.
- **Create routine** by getting the kids to help make a weekly planner with colour-coded activities, so they know exactly what to do and when. Make sure it has a good mix of activities; maybe online classes, study time, reading, leisure time, and household chores like cleaning out a pet's cage or a fish tank. This is structure with empathy built in, because the kids get to have a say in their weekly schedule and can take ownership of getting the tasks done.
- **Stay active.** Find ways to keep active safely. That might mean indoors if the weather is bad or it's not a safe environment outside your home. Sites like gonoodle.com are great, and you can find plenty of other fun activities to try on sites like

YouTube Kids.

- **Take breaks.** Kids don't sit at their desks all day at school, so remember to build in snack time, recess, lunch, and allow space to change mindset between 'classes'. During breaks, have a change in scene where possible, by going for a walk, or change to a different activity.

Parenting and homeschooling in a pandemic is hard. You won't be perfect and that's okay. If you can answer the following six questions each day, then that's good enough in the short term while you figure out more sustainable solutions that work for your family.

1. Did everyone learn something new today?
2. Did everyone get a chance to practise something they already know?
3. Is everyone safe?
4. Is everyone fed?
5. Did we all make it through the day okay given all the stresses we are experiencing right now?
6. What could we do differently tomorrow?

Let's talk about screen time

With so many of us now working from home and a high chance that you have spent, or are still spending, a lot of time trying to homeschool your kids, it's likely your household rules around screen time slipped long ago.

Screen time recommendations come from a variety of sources, including the World Health Organization, the American Academy of Pediatrics, and the Australian Government Department of Health. All of them say that children aged two to five probably shouldn't have more than one hour of screen time per day, ideally watching with an adult. Guidelines for school-aged children are looser, because the appropriate amount of screen time is considered to depend on the lifestyle of the child. This leaves it up to parents to figure out what's best.

For kids and adults alike, this new way of living and working has revealed how much time we really spend in front of screens and some of us don't like what we see. Experts tell us that it's fine to be more flexible about the time your kids are spending online right now, providing you use effective parental controls, protect them from digital risks and stop them using their devices in the bedroom. But is that really happening in your household? And what kind of screen time are you clocking up these days, with all that Zoom and Netflix time, and checking through Twitter, Facebook and Instagram?

Screen time is also a really important means for us to be able to do our work and keep the kids occupied, so how do we strike the balance? How much is too much, and is all screen time the same anyway?

If we look closely at the recommendations, then there are three common factors that underpin healthy technology use for children (and adults too): time, quality, and relationships.

1. Time spent in front of a screen. The impact of technology on children's health, wellbeing, social and emotional outcomes and their school achievement too depends less on the amount of time spent in front of a screen and more on the type of content they engage with when using a screen.

2. The quality of the content you are engaging with. Passive screen time, things like watching TV or scrolling through your Instagram feed, is usually associated with the negative effects like depression, moodiness, anxiety, and physical inactivity. Active screen time, stuff that engages you physically or cognitively, can actually be helpful.

3. Relationships. Who are you using the screen with? When used wisely, screens also allow us to stay connected with people through technology like FaceTime and Zoom. While social media comes with risks of overwhelm due to drama, trolls or pressure to make ourselves look good to others, in many studies a majority of teens say that social media helps the relationships they already have with their friends.

Being online can also help you find your tribe, through tools like multiplayer video games, Twitch streams, or Reddit. If you don't quite fit in where you live or you live in a small or isolated community, quality screen time might be essential to keeping you well.

For kids and teens, healthy screen use is all about striking a balance between these three factors, time, quality, and relationships. The best quality content is interactive, age-appropriate, educational and encourages children to persevere when they strike a problem. There aren't too many bells and whistles to bait your child into continued use, nor in-app purchases that not only hit you in the wallet, but encourage your child to take the short cut to the solution rather than put the effort in.

Co-viewing, where a child uses a screen with a parent who can explain ideas to them, can be a positive way to build relationships with screen time. You may also hear the term co-engaging when talking about older children. This means using a screen with someone equally as engaged, such as playing an online game with a parent or friend, or taking part in a virtual study group on Skype.

If you suspect — or know — that your child may have fallen into using a screen for longer periods because of all the changes brought by the coronavirus, then try to ensure screen quality and screen relationships are taken into account.

Set up time to engage in a screen activity with your child and look for a quality educational experience that you can do together. These questions can help you decide whether the app offers an engaging learning experience for you and your child:

1. Does the platform or app excite the senses? By stimulating their senses, the app will be more likely to provide physical and mental challenges that promote higher order thinking through the combination of curiosity and self-motivated learning that spur memory and reasoning activity.

2. Will your child connect with the content? Is it familiar to them? Are the characters and style of the app relevant to their preferences and daily life? Using apps that combine familiar characters and themes is far more likely to keep your child engaged and excited about learning.

3. Does the app tell a story that continues to keep your child engaged? A good app will track your child's progress and progressively present more challenging content to create a positive learning experience.

4. Does the app encourage social interaction? Look out for interactive tasks and shared learning; perhaps there's a character that needs help on a journey, or maybe needs two or three users to work together at a time. Apps like this can help promote skills in teamwork, leadership and problem-solving.

How to support kids through Covid-19

- **Reassure** them they are safe.
- **Encourage** them to talk about how they feel.
- **Tell them they can ask questions,** and answer these in plain language appropriate to their age — be honest but avoid details that may distress or cause anxiety. Don't force it — if your child is getting distressed in the conversation you're having about Covid-19, then reassure them and end it. You can come back to it another time when they might be more ready.
- **Tell them that feeling upset or afraid is normal,** that it's good to talk about it and that they'll feel better soon.
- **Be understanding.** They may have problems sleeping, throw tantrums or wet the bed — be patient and reassuring if this happens. With support and care, it will pass.
- **Give your children extra love and attention.** It's okay to spoil them a bit with that right now. All children really need is a full tummy, a safe space and, most of all, love from their parents.
- **Remember that children look to their parents to feel safe and to know how to respond.** Reassure them, share that you are upset too but that you know you will all be fine together. And if you're finding things hard, that's common — these are extraordinary circumstances and you're doing your best. If you need support, please don't be afraid to reach out — all of us need help sometimes.
- **If you're in lockdown,** work as a team and use the Five Ways to Wellbeing to map out what a day might look like. The Five Ways means consciously adding activities that enable you to connect, give, take notice, keep learning and be active. I recommend you try to throw in five doses

of fun as well. It sounds like a big ask, but these moments are great little mood flippers and circuit breakers that can really lift everyone's spirits, boost connection and help your kids move from one emotional state to another.

- **Finally, try to keep to normal routines** like mealtime and bedtimes. Allow them to burn off their energy as much as you can, and as restrictions allow.

Pre-teens, teens and social media

For older kids, social media presents additional screen-time challenges. Parents rightly worry about time spent on social media and perhaps online bullying too. Encourage your teens to get off social media and connecting through apps that allow video calls like FaceTime and WhatsApp so they can connect one to one.

This pandemic is especially hard for teens because just at a time that they want to be spreading their wings, experimenting and discovering things about themselves and the world, they are being required to stay at home. At a time when their peer relationships are becoming some of the most important in their lives, they're being asked to pare this back and spend more time with their family. To them, that seems pretty unfair, and I think that's fair enough.

Listening to their protestations and railing against the unfairness of it all won't change the situation, but it will help them to see that you understand, and perhaps help you all plan for what they might be able to do when the situation becomes safe again. This is also an opportunity for you to reinforce how important it is for everyone to play their part, and how that involves sacrifices for many of us right now.

Gen Z

The pandemic has clipped the wings of our young adults too, those late teenagers and early 20-somethings who should be emerging into the world of work and career and adulthood, at this time of incredible uncertainty. How can we help Generation Z (those born after 1997) navigate this crisis, when so much of what they hoped and planned for has been wrenched from their grasp through no fault of their own?

Here I think it's helpful to consider the lessons from Gail Sheehy's influential book, *Passages: Predictable Crises of Adult Life*. This book was first published in 1976, when I was seven years old, and has since been named one of the 10 most influential books by the US Library of Congress. When I was an undergraduate student, this book made a lasting impression on me, and I think it's worth reflecting on Sheehy's work to make sense of some of our Covid-19 pandemic experiences, particularly those of young adults.

In every culture there are expected life transitions or 'passages', like graduating or entering the world of work, setting up an independent home or having children. As a society or a culture, we have an expected trajectory of how and when these things will unfold, and an individual's expectations of how and when these passages will unfold are often shaped by the experiences of peers or older siblings. Any sense of being 'off-time' with these 'passages' can be experienced as a sense that one is failing, or being left behind.

Even before this pandemic, many of the millennial generation were experiencing lives that felt 'off-time' from the norms expected of them. Many continue to live at home into their twenties and thirties, and a large proportion are neither working nor in education, meaning that they are essentially held back from passages towards their next stages of adult development, increasing this sense of feeling 'off-time'. They can't even begin to think about goals like saving money to buy a house, getting married, formally entering into a long-term stable relationship, or any kind of career security.

The passage into adulthood has never been easy, but right now it seems especially fraught and difficult. In previous generations the threats were external: wars, communism, and the nuclear bomb. Today, for many young people, the enemies are internal: drugs, guns, and violence.

Enter the Covid-19 pandemic, and we can see this strain may be amplified. The life events that mark moving away from your family of origin have morphed into something else, or have disappeared completely. Many are having to move back to family homes because the world has changed in such a way that independence has become much more difficult to secure.

In New Zealand, a generation of children who started school when the Canterbury earthquake sequence was at its most active are now young people leaving the schooling system. In the US, a generation of children born in the aftermath of 9/11 and raised in the shadow of school shootings are now graduating into a transforming working world of a global pandemic and possibly the deepest economic depression in living memory.

Developing their internal system for motivation and drive is going to be critical for Gen Z. Unless we help them to navigate through these times, unless we force open the door of opportunity for them to progress in the real world, there is a very real danger that they are likely to feel their motivation start to slip away.

Young graduates were already finding it difficult to get jobs out of university or college, and now competition for jobs in a depressed economy will increase. Indeed, there may be a sense that people are educated for jobs that may be even harder to get than they were before, placing pressure on education systems to understand future needs in a post-pandemic world.

Repeated and persistent failure to progress and succeed in a world where their opportunities may become severely limited could generate learned helplessness on an epic scale. Already, we are seeing our youngest generations reporting high levels of stress and poor mental health. We need to be especially mindful if we are not to strip this generation of its motivation to try again once opportunities start to emerge.

But just as difficult life events also offer the potential to emerge stronger, more resilient, and more committed to a set of values that help us to navigate future difficult circumstances, so might Covid-19 prove a similarly testing and resilience-building stressor.

Sheehy calls the first stage of adult learning the Tryout Twenties, a time when we try out different roles in work and in relationships. But what if the usual opportunities for learning that we go through in our twenties are overtaken by the pandemic? It's hard to learn to compete and cooperate in jobs when they are scarce, or when collaboration has become a logistical dance of internet connection and physical distancing. It's challenging to make and maintain new relationships when it's difficult to get around the country or meet in person for romantic trysts.

The new rites of passage for this generation might look different and require different skill sets, but they remain challenges all the same and still demand both motivation and compassion.

Sheehy sees the outbreak of caring that we have seen in these pandemic times as more than a match for the voracious all-consuming appetite of the virus. We have seen this in the stories of doctors and nurses who have isolated themselves from their families for weeks at a time so they can assist on the frontline, sometimes sacrificing their lives to care for the needs of others. We have seen this in the caring choices of many to stay away from their vulnerable loved ones, to shield them from the risk of being infected by the virus, sometimes not knowing if they will ever see their ageing parents again.

In this time, it is more important than ever to mourn these losses, of contact, of rituals like funerals and weddings, of events that mark the passages into different phases of life. This time too will pass. The toll is cumulative, but we will adapt. We will find new rituals, and new passages into the next stage of life.

We live among generations who have no memory of a pre-internet world, who have no idea of what the 'Cold War' means. In 1994, we had no idea how internet-dependent life would become. Into 1985, we had no idea what a post-USSR world might look like, and the tortuous changes to global geopolitics that would follow, and how this also clashed and became entangled with our internet dependency.

So, as we remain rightly concerned about lost opportunities for Generation Z, and perhaps ourselves depending on our circumstances and life stage, remember that we are social beings who would not have survived as a species were it not for the fact that we care for each other.

As Sheehy herself has said, perhaps it won't only be smart thinking that helps us to emerge from these pandemic times. 'I care, therefore I am.' What might emerge from these pandemic times is an increasing realisation that those communities that coped best were those with a sensitivity and empathy towards their own and others' experiences.

It is this connection with our own experience and towards our fellow travellers on this planet that might be the defining outcome, determining who is best placed to move forwards. It might just be that Generation Z, with the knowledge of the importance of the balance between what we think, how we feel, and how these are intertwined, become our guides and leaders when we exit into whatever is yet to come.

CHAPTER 7

Access to quality information

On 4 April 2020, a *Los Angeles Times* story about the varying effects of the novel coronavirus contained a fascinating paragraph:

'One thing to keep in mind before we continue: It is possible that the information you read below will be contradicted in the coming weeks or that gaps in knowledge today will soon be filled as scientists continue to study the virus.'

The paragraph was interesting because the *Los Angeles Times* was admitting that its information was incomplete and subject to revision. News organisations and others intent on projecting authority and knowledge (such as government spokespersons) rarely admit their fallibility or lack of omniscience.

The paragraph goes to the heart of one of the great challenges of this pandemic: getting access to quality information.[1] In reality, all information is provisional, not final. Knowing that the information is likely to change does not mean it isn't true; that's simply the nature of scientific understanding. As new data becomes available, there's a likelihood that it changes your understanding of the situation.

---

1. https://www.pressclubinstitute.org/a-caveat-how-an-la-times-science-writer-explains-coronavirus-uncertainty/

In the early days, when we knew reasonably little about the pandemic virus and how it was likely to affect us, there was much new data, and our understanding shifted a lot. This doesn't mean that our previous understanding was false or untrue. It was simply the best we could do with the data at that time.

The same pattern continues as we journey forwards. More data becomes available on the lasting impacts of Covid-19, how easily it is transmitted in particular circumstances, and how the vaccine efforts are progressing through various clinical trials, and so our understanding is updated.

The problem of the internet age is that the information already out there doesn't get erased when new data comes to light that may change our understanding. The challenge for individuals is to take on new information and to refresh and update our understanding of how it may affect our lives.

The challenge for journalists and politicians is to communicate information in a way that makes it clear that the current understanding is provisional and subject to change. Politicians and officials must be confident and firm enough to recommend actions based on this information that both maximise the possibility of safety and security, while minimising the risks of unintended harm, such as severe economic damage. It is not an easy balance to strike and it will not be ending any time soon, but as has been said many, many times over in this pandemic, there is no economy without people.

What's important is that we can trust each other that when decisions need to be made, they are made transparently and on the basis of information that is available for all to see. And that's where our leaders have an important role to play.

Information from official sources

From community groups to the highest levels of government, we rely on our leaders to guide us in uncertain times.

We need them to help us understand the threat and what's at stake. Even where information may be subject to future change, we need them to offer clear advice to help us keep ourselves and others safe. We need to understand why we are being asked to take these actions and how they might affect us in the future. And most of all, we need recognition for the difficulties and hardships we may face in following the official advice or complying with restrictions. In other words, we need both structure and empathy from our leaders.

Leaders can provide structure by creating well thought out and helpful guidelines, rather than hasty policy responses. A good example is the four-level Covid-19 alert system rolled out by the New Zealand Government in March 2020. At that time the disease was present in the country but had not yet become widespread.

The alert system laid out four levels of restrictions that would be applied, depending on the spread of the disease within the community. If the disease was contained (level 1), life would carry on more or less as normal (minus the international travel), with increased emphasis on precautions like hand washing and keeping a record of movements. As disease is transmitted in the community (level 2), the risk of spread increases (level 3) or if outbreaks become widespread (level 4), different levels of restrictions would come into force, such as the closures of schools, restaurants and recreational facilities, a restriction on the maximum size for any gathering, or full 'lockdown'.

By clearly stating the restrictions at each alert level and explaining the reasons for those restrictions, the government gave strong signals of what might happen in the future. This meant the public had a good idea of what to expect and why, which brought some helpful predictability to an uncertain situation. When lockdown restrictions were subsequently imposed and later eased, the public had a framework to help them understand the reasons why.

But there was one crucial factor that ensured the effectiveness of this system: empathy. When New Zealand's four-level alert system was announced, and on subsequent occasions when the system was referred to or alert level changes were imposed, the Prime Minister Jacinda Ardern acknowledged that these restrictions would be challenging for some, but urged the country to pull together as a 'team of five million' to protect the most vulnerable.

When structure is imposed without empathy, we can feel stifled or restricted and we can be tempted to rebel even when we know the advice is in service of a greater good. If we end up with mixed messaging, and different strategies operating at the same time, this leads to more confusion, uncertainty and anxiety, hampering the ability to create a cohesive response.

In contrast, when leaders offer well thought out and helpful structures, delivered with clear and empathetic communication, this engages our personal internal drive system, so we can find the motivation to do what we need to do no matter how hard it might be. It also creates a sense of being in this together, which can help us do well in a crisis.

Developing this sort of policy response requires both creative and strategic thinking — and that is only possible if our leaders can master their internal systems too. As you'll recall from chapter 1, strategic and creative thinking is very much dependent on being able to get out of threat detection mode, and being able to engage our internal system of calming and engaging with our values in order to come up with more reasoned and strategic thinking.

Structure and empathy comes from internal systems mastery. Internal systems mastery comes from structure and empathy.

If you're leading a community group or an organisation in a time of crisis, it's important that you use both structure and empathy in your communications. Structure helps to give people clear direction on what they need to do and when, with clear updates and transparency when the situation changes, and with all leaders operating and sticking to the same framework and messages. Empathy recognises that these directions can be difficult for people to put into practice in their lives, and may involve offering practical advice and guidance, or thanking your team when they take the recommended actions.

As much as possible, try to be empathetic and helpful in your planning and design work, and in your use of language, because this is how you create a sense of being 'all in this together'. All people really want to know is what's the right thing to do, whether they're doing it, and if it is working. Simply acknowledging their efforts can go a long way towards generating support for your plan. This builds a much more sustainable response, likely to carry a greater proportion of people forwards, for the greatest amount of time. And this momentum is critically important to keep people going through the toughest times.

The phenomenon of social proof

The trouble is, not all of the official information has been delivered in this way — far from it. Depending where you live, you may have been given conflicting information by different government agencies. You may have seen restrictions change over time or even at short notice, without clear explanation of the reasons for the change. And we've all seen advice about keeping yourself safe from the virus change, as evidence and understanding has developed over time. As *New York Times* opinion writer Charlie Warzel pointed out, the official advice about wearing masks changed completely in the course of a month.[2]

The question about masks is just one rapidly shifting element among a wide-ranging group of stories whose facts are updated daily, if not hourly. This pandemic is not a one-day story like a press conference or a fire. It is an ongoing story made up of a series of events, public statements, investigative reports, research findings, political decisions and other facts that emerge all the time. Each of these adds to, and changes, the gathering rolling stone of truth.

These constantly shifting sands are confusing and wearying for people, and especially difficult to process in uncertain situations. When we are feeling unsure, we look to people we trust and respect to figure out the 'correct' way to behave. This is a phenomenon known as social proof and it is driven by an assumption that others in your network know more about a situation than you do. It is also part of our evolutionary programming: in uncharted territory it's best to stick with the herd and move with the herd, lest we become an outlier, too slow to respond, and get picked off by the predator.

Whether in online communities like Facebook groups, on other social media like Instagram, or in real life, the amount of similarity a person or group might have to you is an important influence. A person who is ambivalent and may be persuadable is more likely to adopt behaviour and attitudes of people who are perceived to be similar to themselves, and are therefore seen to be easy to relate to. Research on social proof has shown that our peers, in particular,

2. https://www.nytimes.com/2020/07/22/opinion/coronavirus-health-experts.html

and their choices are important to us and influence our decisions and actions: we usually choose to do the same thing that our peers are doing.

Social proof becomes more influential when the surrounding people are perceived as particularly knowledgeable about a situation or are even just slightly more familiar with the situation than the observer is. And this is all about perception — that familiarity doesn't even have to be based in fact. The engine of social proof works best when the proof is provided by the behaviour and actions of a larger number of people. It seems that the greater the number of people or 'agencies' who find an idea to be correct, the more correct and valid the idea will be for the ambiguous and persuadable observer.

When you consider that about 30% of US adults think that the coronavirus was created and spread on purpose and that the threat of Covid-19 has been exaggerated to damage Donald Trump, then you can see why these ideas can spread quite quickly, and can potentially be very damaging such as when people won't wear masks in a pandemic or refuse to comply with contact tracing information requests.

Social proof can be useful in a teaching context, as kids can learn academic and prosocial skills by watching each other. It's also used by therapists in treating phobias. Children who are afraid of dogs can quickly overcome their fear by watching another child play happily with a dog, or even watching videos of other children playing with dogs. The observing child still knows that dogs can be dangerous, but that fear is now overwritten with social proof that dogs must be safe.

In an internet-dominated world, social proof gets messy. Whatever catches your attention on your social media and internet feeds like Google, Facebook, Instagram, YouTube and Twitter, has first go at influencing your behaviour. And the algorithms that determine what shows up in your social media and internet feeds are only partly based on your unique browsing and clicking history. You're also being served up whatever content is getting clicks and attracting watch time on various social media channels and platforms.

What it comes down to is this: internet and social media platforms want to sell you things. In order to sell you things, they need to show you lots of targeted advertising. And to create opportunities to show you advertising, they will show you content that will keep you watching for a longer period of time. And the more weird, extreme or polarising the content, the longer we tend to watch, which means they can show you more ads, and convert your attention to sales.

Given that in uncertain situations we like to take the lead from those who we already know, imagine that your friend has just liked or shared a piece of content that was weird or extreme enough to get them engaged. The algorithms then proceed to place this in your feed, because you are part of your friend's network. And because you respect your friend's opinion, consciously or not, you engage with this new content, whether you click on it or not. Even lingering as you scroll by is registered by the social media platforms as a form of positive engagement, making it more likely that you will be served with similar content again.

Little by little, as you view this content, more extreme ideas about the pandemic, where it came from and how best to deal with it become ever so slightly more normalised through sheer familiarity. Your brain makes the connection that if your own network seems to be giving these ideas validity, then everyone else must be too. This is also how attitudes get changed, and how we are shaped by what our social networks are showing us.

Once we become aware of this, as many of us are now doing, it's tempting to wall ourselves off and make decisions based upon our own hunches because we conclude that our guess is as good as anybody else's. In most cases, though, when we are looking at public health threats, it isn't. Our risk-averse tendency in uncertain times may cause us to throw the proverbial baby out with the bathwater.

It's hard to maintain trust in experts when they're struggling to piece things together too. But it's also highly likely that, although mistakes may be made along the way, the experts have more up to date and useful information than the polarising opinion pieces and Facebook group posts promoted by the revenue-driven algorithms on your phone.

So, yes, it's fatiguing to keep on top of things, and it's tempting to bury your head in the sand or fall for simple solutions and explanations which help you to live in a simpler world away from the complex reality we find ourselves in. But at what cost?

The lives and livelihoods of those we care most dearly about, the communities we grew up in, the neighbourhoods we live in, the companies and organisations we work in and may have built up ourselves. There is too much at stake to stay divorced from reality for too long, though who can blame us for wanting respite from the sheer unrelenting horror and paralysing monotony of it all?

Practising discernment

Access to quality information — and knowing how to discern the quality of the information — is an essential part of citizenship in a democracy. These days we are bombarded with news articles, blogs, posts on Facebook, videos on YouTube from a variety of sources, some credible, some not so credible, and some with outright ulterior motives. It's hard to know who and what to trust.

With so much information coming at us, it's important to only consume what you can handle. Of course you should keep up with the news so that you can protect yourself and others; everyone needs to strike a balance between remaining informed and giving the scary stuff too much attention. When we feel overwhelmed by what's happening in the world, we can be more likely to feel anxious.

If you're having a tough time or a hard day, you don't have to keep watching live news, use social media, or allow notifications on your phone. Instead, make a conscious decision to limit the time you spend reading or watching things which aren't making you feel better. Be strict with yourself and make a commitment that you will only watch the news or read an update on the virus once a day. This can ease anxiety by reducing the amount of time you think about it or absorbing new information about a difficult situation.

The same goes for social media. Social media can be a brilliant tool for staying connected with friends, family and the wider world. During the initial lockdowns, Facebook Messenger use for group calls surged by as much as 70 percent.[3] It also doesn't take much mental discipline and that can be appealing in alarming times. When it's hard to concentrate on anything else, many of us will take the easy option and veg out with some mindless scrolling.

But we also know that social media has a dark side. Since it's a relatively new technology, little is known about the long-term consequences of social media use. However, multiple studies have

---

3. https://www.cnet.com/news/facebook-sees-surge-of-engagement-worldwide-following-coronavirus-outbreak/

found a strong link between heavy social media and an increased risk for depression, anxiety, loneliness, self-harm, and even suicidal thoughts.[4] Those are the last things we need when we're dealing with a deadly disease and possibly staying at home, grieving for lost normalcy or feeling anticipatory grief over future lost lives.

So why does something that can be so positive and fuel connection have such capacity to bring us down and provoke these reactions in our behavioural immune systems? There's a real similarity between emotions and viruses. Both can be contagious in real life, but whereas viruses can't be caught online, emotions can — in a very real way. As we've already seen, social media algorithms amplify and spread the most intense posts so that we all get exposed. As our social media feeds turn into a flurry of anxiety, fear and anger, there's a risk of escalating and spreading these feelings via retweets and likes.

You didn't have to spend long on social media after the onset of the Covid-19 pandemic to find that the general vibe was distinctly negative. According to marketing companies that tracked these things, feelings of fear and disgust rose along with the number of posts.

This is important when we consider what has been called the behavioural immune system. Mark Schaller at the University of British Columbia in Vancouver came up with this concept of a set of unconscious psychological responses designed to act as a first line of defence to reduce our contact with potential harmful viruses and bacteria.[5] The evolutionary advantage here is that anything

4. For example: Phu, B & Gow, AJ (2019). Facebook use and its association with subjective happiness and loneliness. *Computers in Human Behavior.* 92:151–159.
5. Schaller, M (2011). The behavioural immune system and the psychology of human

that reduces the risk of infection should offer a distinct survival advantage.

The disgust response seems to be a fundamental element of the behavioural immune system. When we avoid things that smell bad or food we believe to be tainted somehow, we are instinctively trying to avoid potential contagion. Just the merest suggestion that we have already eaten something rotten can cause us to vomit, hopefully ejecting the food before the infection has a chance to take hold. Research also suggests that we also tend to more strongly remember material that triggers disgust, allowing us to remember (and avoid) the situations that could put us at risk of infection later on.

Schaller argues that many of our social rules or norms — such as the ways we should and should not prepare food, the amount of social contact that is and isn't accepted, or how to dispose of human waste — can help to reduce the risk of infection. Schaller suggests that people who conform to those norms serve a public health service, and people who violate those norms not only put themselves at risk, but affect others as well. As a result, it's beneficial to become more respectful of convention in the face of a contagious outbreak. This is why it's so important to build new norms and reinforce them alongside helpful existing norms in the face of a pandemic threat.

The flip side is that the behavioural immune system may make us more distrustful of strangers, and also perhaps shape our responses to people of different cultural backgrounds. According to Schaller, this may arise from those fears about non-conformity: in the past, people outside our group may have been less likely to

sociality. *Philosophical Transactions of the Royal Society of London*. Series B, Biological sciences, 366(1583), 3418–3426. https://doi.org/10.1098/rstb.2011.0029

observe the specific prescriptive norms that were meant to protect the population from infection, so we feared that they would unwittingly (or deliberately) spread disease. Today we see that it can result in racism, prejudice and xenophobia, with all the resulting hysteria about bat-eating, pangolin traders and other extreme reactions on social media. In one sense, we can frame this as a behavioural immune system response designed to protect us. But if we take a rational step back, we can perhaps see this in another way: a response that creates division, misunderstanding and prejudice at a time when there has never been a greater need to work together to find a way to neutralise the threat of Covid-19.

For all these reasons, and to cut this long story short, I recommend we all practise social media distancing, and set ourselves some rules. *It's fine to check Facebook — but make it once or twice a day. It's okay to check Twitter, but not after 9pm.* Quarantine your social media to prevent it from infecting your whole day.

Social media apps are designed to be addictive, so I don't recommend going cold turkey. You'll find it easier if you intentionally replace it with something else that is distracting, rewarding and useful. Instead of using the apps on your phone, why not use the phone for its legacy features? Make a phone call instead and enjoy the benefits of real connection.

CHAPTER 8

Conspiracy theories

Whether we know it or not, when we engage online we are constantly encountering misinformation, disinformation and conspiracy theories. These are all subtly different, but they have a common theme of untrue information competing for space with verified facts. This means that what we need to do in order to stay well or make good decisions can get lost in all the noise we are trying to filter and process.

Many of these posts are designed to catch attention with shocking headlines or 'statistics'. On social media we often move quickly, skimming information, and not necessarily stopping to check the source. With the ease of clicking 'Like' and 'Share', it's all too easy for you or others you love to unwittingly playing a role in amplifying disinformation, misinformation or conspiracy theories.

The bad news is that whether this is done by mistake or by people actively spreading and recruiting others to do the same, false information can seriously affect our way of life, our democracy, our health, and our economies.

And during the Covid-19 pandemic, it has been spreading, fast. Our need for structure in uncertain times, combined with our pattern recognition skills, can become overactive, creating a tendency to spot patterns —like constellations, clouds that look like dogs and vaccines causing autism — where in fact there is none.

The ability to see patterns was a useful survival trait for our ancestors. It's far better to mistakenly spot signs of a predator than to overlook a hungry predator. But put the same tendency in our information-rich world and we start to see non-existent links between cause and effect — otherwise known as conspiracy theories — all over the place.

So what is a conspiracy theory? According to Joseph Uscinski, Associate Professor of Political Science at the University of Miami, a conspiracy theory 'is an accusatory perception in which a small group of powerful people are working in secret for their own benefit against the common good and in a way that undermines our bedrock ground rules against widespread force and fraud, and that perception has yet to be verified by the appropriate experts using available and open data and methods'.[1] If this sounds like a complicated description to you, you're right: it does to me too. A simpler working definition for this book could be the idea that certain events or trends are the products of deceptive plots that are largely unknown to the general public.

Conspiracy theories are nothing new. A University of Chicago study estimated in 2014 that half of the American public consistently endorses at least one conspiracy theory. Further studies have shown that people are likely to turn to conspiracy theories when they are anxious and feel powerless. Other research indicates that conspiracy theory belief is strongly related to lack of sociopolitical control or lack of psychological empowerment.

Among many other reasons, belief in conspiracy theory also appears to be partly predicted by the perception that society is under threat, and that society's fundamental values are changing. A lack of control over perception of these changes can lead to people

1. Quoted from: Why Your Brain Loves Conspiracy Theories by Robert Roy Britt, 8 September 2020: https://elemental.medium.com/why-your-brain-loves-conspiracy-theories-69ca2abd893a

to exaggerate the influence that they attribute to their 'enemies', and can deepen their belief in conspiracies, provided that the perceivers consider the implicated authorities or 'enemies' as immoral.

Conspiracy theories do not seem to be restricted to specific times or cultures: citizens around the world are susceptible to them, from modern to traditional societies. The tendency to be suspicious of the possibility that others are forming conspiracies against one and one's group may well be a fundamental part of human nature.

One reason why we are so keen to believe in conspiracy theories is that we are social animals. From an evolutionary standpoint, our status in society is much more important than being right, so we constantly compare our actions and beliefs to those of our peers, and then alter them to fit in. This means that if our social group believes something, we are more likely to follow the herd.

The principle applies powerfully to ideas. As we've seen with social proof, the more people who believe a piece of information, then the more likely we are to accept it as true. If we are overly exposed to a particular idea through our social group, whether on social media or in real life, then that becomes embedded in our world view. In fact, social proof is a much more effective persuasion technique than purely evidence-based proof, which is why we see it so often in advertising. If '80% of mums agree', then the product must be good, right?

Another logical fallacy that causes us to overlook information is confirmation bias, that tendency for people to seek out and believe the data that supports their views while discounting the stuff that doesn't. We all suffer from this. Just think back to the last time you heard a debate on the radio or television. How convincing did you find the argument that ran counter to your view compared to the one that agreed with it?

The chances are that, whatever the rationality of either side, you largely dismissed the opposition arguments while applauding those who agreed with you. Confirmation bias also shows itself as a tendency to select information from sources that already agree with our views (which probably comes from the social group that we relate to). Hence your political beliefs probably dictate your preferred news outlets.

So what can you do when you encounter misinformation and conspiracy theories online, or perhaps shared and endorsed by friends and loved ones? Taking a myth-busting approach might seem like a good way to go. Perhaps calling out the myth and then presenting reality seems like a logical, fact-based way to present corrective information so people can change their behaviour, based on good evidence. The truth will always win, right?

Unfortunately, this is not how the brain with its inherent cognitive biases paired with social influences works. What it actually seems to do is trigger what has become known as the backfire effect, where the myth ends up becoming more memorable than the fact. In a study evaluating a 'Myths and Facts' flyer about flu vaccines, things seemed to go well initially. Immediate after reading the flyer, study participants accurately remembered the facts as facts and myths as myths. But only 30 minutes later, this completely changed, with myths becoming much more likely to be remembered as 'facts'.[2]

It seems as though merely mentioning the myths actually seems to reinforce them. And then over time — and a shockingly short period of time at that — you forget the context in which you heard the myth. Even in the context of a myth-debunking flyer, the participant

2. Memory for Flu Facts and Myths and Effects on Vaccine Intentions: https://clinicaltrials.gov/ct2/show/record/NCT00296270

is more likely to be left with just the memory of the myth itself, as fact.

If myth-busting isn't the way to go, what should you do to reduce the spread of misinformation or outright disinformation on the internet through your own social media use? Here are three things to try.

First, only share information you know is factually accurate. Research tells us quite clearly that even if you consider yourself the smartest of people, you can easily be fooled by fake claims because of something called cognitive miserliness. This is the brain's tendency to seek solutions that take the least mental effort. Translation: we don't want to think, and we avoid it at all costs!

We have all formed habits that enable us to virtually bypass the thinking process. We've hardwired our brains to take shortcuts. For many adults, this 'non-thinking' aspect runs on autopilot. It's as if the brain knows no other way, so we must actively guard against it.

The best way to do that is to make sure you're only sharing information from official sources, not obscure things from Twitter, Reddit, or a Facebook post your friend says they *heard from their sister who works in a place where they know a guy who said they saw someone doing something they shouldn't have done, and then this has suddenly caused a massive outbreak of Covid-19 that's being hushed up, and you heard it here first.*

Don't share that kind of thing, because you shouldn't underestimate the power of the social media algorithms to viralise posts that aren't true but produce clicks. Algorithms tend not to care whether the thing you're posting is true or not. And if you're sharing it, then you're not part of the solution — you're part of the problem.

Second, keep your emotions in check. If you do engage and try to debunk a false claim, then try not to get too emotional about it because that makes people who disagree with you much more likely to share the information that you're trying to debunk. And so the spiral continues.

Presenting corrective information to a group with firmly held beliefs can actually strengthen their views, despite the new information undermining it. New evidence creates inconsistencies in our beliefs and an associated emotional discomfort. Instead of modifying our beliefs, we tend to invoke self-justification and even stronger dislike of opposing theories, which can make us more entrenched in our views. This has become known as the as the 'boomerang effect' — and it is a huge problem when trying to nudge people towards better behaviours.

To avoid the backfire or boomerang effects, ignore the myths. Just make the key points: *vaccines are safe and reduce the chances of getting flu by between 50% and 60%,* full stop. Don't mention or acknowledge the misconceptions, as they tend to be better remembered.

Don't get people riled up by challenging their worldview. Instead offer explanations that chime with their pre-existing beliefs. For example, conservative climate-change deniers are much more likely to shift their views if they are also presented with the pro-environment business opportunities.

Work carried out by psychologist Dr Jay Van Bavel shows that using moderate language, rather than polarising language, most likely increases how far your debunking message travels to the people who need to hear it, rather than just bouncing around your own bubble or echo chamber of people who already agree with you. So if you're really trying to address the problem, don't do it for the likes — look beyond that, moderate your language, and don't mention the conspiracy if you can avoid it.

Third, ask questions. If you get into an active disagreement with someone sharing a conspiracy theory, try asking questions rather than simply presenting facts. Ask them to explain how their elaborate conspiracy works, rather than why they believe it. This is important because experiments show that focusing on explaining how the conspiracy works tends to bring home the fact that they don't understand the details of the issue as well as they think they do.

This is called the illusion of explanatory depth. Once you shine a light on how shallow the conspiracy theory actually is, then this seems to be more useful in prompting them to question their beliefs, rather than countering them with facts alone.

The biggest power lies in pre-bunking rather than debunking. That means pre-emptively warning people about the strategies that people are using to speed conspiracy theories, like high-end production values and the use of fake experts. And it's important that we get ahead of this, because it's likely there will be an explosion of conspiracy theories about the safety and effectiveness of Covid-19 vaccines.

A good way to learn about these strategies is with the Bad News online game. It simulates sites like Twitter and allows you to build your follower base by applying misinformation techniques, like impersonating or delegitimising official accounts by attacking them in different ways, making polarising comments designed to create partisan divides, or through creating complete conspiracy theories. By demonstrating techniques like mocking, falsifying, exaggerating, manipulating, frightening, denying and outright lying, it appears to help to insulate people against the effects of disinformation when they encounter it in their real lives and will give you some insight into how to protect yourself and others from disinformation.

You're not going to stop everyone out there spreading misinformation, but like a real virus the survival of misinformation depends on its R, or reproduction number. We all need to play our part in stopping the spread of the Covid-19 infodemic — and actually any other conspiracy theory you come across. If we can get enough people not to pass the misinformation virus on, then we might be able to reduce its spread and at least get it under control, even if we can't completely eliminate it.

How to fact check

According to Michael Lynch, a professor of philosophy at the University of Connecticut, the internet is both the best fact-checking device that humanity could have invented and the best bias-confirming device that we could have invented.[3]

The key to making thoughtful decisions is to use the power of the internet to check your facts instead of turning it into an echo chamber for beliefs you already hold. Professor Sam Wineburg of Stanford University has researched the techniques used by professional fact checkers at some of the world's most prestigious publications and discovered they use a very different approach when landing on an unfamiliar website.

Most of us — including academics, students and thoughtful adults — tend to read a web page from top to bottom and back again,

3. Lynch, MP (2017). *The Internet of Us: Knowing More and Understanding Less in the Age of Big Data*. Liveright.

in the same way that we would read a printed document.[4] Professional fact checkers read horizontally, which means that when they hit an unfamiliar website they almost immediately open up multiple tabs, working across different pages of the site to get a sense of the organisation that is providing the information. They want to understand and assess the source before they start absorbing the content.

Fact checkers take the website itself with a grain of salt. Anyone can write whatever they want on the website and an 'About' page may not tell the whole story, like who owns the company or who might have influence on the editorial content. Be prepared to dig a little deeper to find out who is really behind the organisation sharing that information.

When researching a website, one of the most useful sources of data can be found in its domain registration details. Over the course of your investigation, it might be relevant to know who — whether it is an organisation or an individual — owns a particular domain, when it was registered and by which registrar, as well as other details. In many cases, this information can be accessed through third-party services such as Whois.

Many of us assume that the higher a page ranks on Google, the more trustworthy the source of information. But that's not always the case. Google ranking is not in itself a seal of approval. Search engine optimisation is complex business and easily manipulated by savvy minds, especially when money is at stake.

When you're trying to check the credibility of a source, pop the name into Google and look beyond the first page to the third, fourth

4. Summarised from my interview with Professor Wineburg on my podcast series *Who Cares? What's the Point?*

or even fifth page of results. According to Moz (a search engine optimisation, or SEO, company), the first page of Google captures 71% of search traffic clicks and has been reported to be as high as 92% in recent years. Second-page results are far from a close second, coming in at below 6% of all website clicks.

So, how do you get on that first page of Google Search results? Often, it's organisations that have paid SEO experts to optimise their content to show up higher in the results. In essence, they are gaming the system in perfectly legitimate ways, but it might not be the best content for your needs. At worst, it is deliberately placed misinformation designed to appear high up in search rankings for popular search terms. And this can be particularly important to bear in mind when searching for information on polarising, contentious topics, where people may be looking to insert their information into other people's social feeds through paid SEO optimisation.

So we can see that getting into pages 3 and 4 of Google Search results might reveal an entirely different take on topics that might seem very different to the information offered in those first two pages. Information consumer, beware ...

Finally, teach your kids about the importance of scrutinising their sources. When you were a student, perhaps you went to the library to do your research. Depending on your age, you may have waded through catalogues, microfiches or indexes to find articles in journals. We'd ask librarians to help us find reputable sources of information.

These days, even at high school, much research is carried out online. Teaching your kids not to take everything at face value and to do their own research before adopting a theory is a vital skill in the Information Age. Young people may be fluent in social media and apps, but that doesn't mean they can easily discern the source of the information.

Another useful site is The Reporters' Lab at Duke University,[5] which maintains a database of global fact-checking sites. You can use their map to check out sites around the world.

Assessing the risks

So how do we assess the risks for ourselves and others, in the face of all this misinformation? What tricks is your mind playing on you to make you consider taking shortcuts, or wiggle around the rules?

Let's start with optimism bias. Optimism bias, sometimes referred to as 'unrealistic optimism', refers to our tendency to underestimate the probability of experiencing adverse effects (such as failure or getting cancer) despite the evidence. Like it or not, most of us carry a little bit of bravado in us, a false confidence that things like car accidents and tragedies happen to 'other' people, not to us. This allows us to keep operating in the world without feeling paralysed by fear, but it can leave us feeling less at risk than we really are, and therefore more willing to take risks.

Another way of looking at it is that optimism bias is the difference between our feeling of hope and reality — humans tend to be predisposed to feeling hope. There's nothing wrong with hope. But it can become a problem when hope makes us lose track of reality and overestimate our chances of success, when the possibility of failure means some pretty high stakes.

How does this happen? Well, the human brain is essentially a

5. https://reporterslab.org/

machine built for jumping to conclusions. Jumping to conclusions can be efficient *if* the conclusions are likely to be correct, the costs of an occasional mistake are acceptable, and if the jump saves much time and effort.

Jumping to conclusions is risky when the situation is unfamiliar, the stakes are high, and there is no time to collect more information, or there is a lag before we can gather more information. That's the situation of this pandemic.

So, how does the brain do this? Think of the brain as broadly having two systems:

- System 1 is about your gut reaction or intuitive thinking. It is fast and about images, emotions, intuition and impressions — it operates automatically and quickly, with little or no effort and no sense of voluntary control.
- System 2 represents the slow, logical and rational; it's analytical thinking — it allocates attention to the effortful mental activities that demand it.

One of the tasks of the analytical thinking system is to overcome the impulses of your gut reactions. In other words, System 2 is in charge of self-control. The best we can do is a compromise: learn to recognise situations in which mistakes are likely and try harder to avoid significant mistakes when the stakes are high by putting analytical thinking in charge.

The trouble is that the effort of will or self-control required to put rational analytical thinking in control is tiring and depleting. If you have to force yourself to do something, you are less willing or less able to exert self-control when the next challenge comes around. This phenomenon is known as ego depletion.

Unlike having just too much stuff to think about at once, ego depletion is at least in part a loss of motivation. After exerting self-control in one task, you do not feel like making an effort in another, although you could do it if you really had to. In several experiments, people were able to resist the effects of ego depletion when given a strong incentive to do so.

So, what's the right incentive? Protecting yourself and others is good, but it might not be enough when we are tired and just want life to go back to how it was. Our brain feels tempted to take the easy way out and become over-optimistic, leading us to take unnecessary risks.

When you feel tempted to 'cheat' the rules, it's time to return to your values. Be aware that your mind will tell you it's okay to fudge the rules a bit, even when it isn't. Put analytical thinking back in charge and stick to who you are.

CHAPTER 9

Coronavirus fatigue

So how is your energy these days? Are you feeling good, full of vital energy? Or are you more depleted and operating on a low level of energy?

If you're feeling more tired than usual or experiencing a general sense of exhaustion, that's understandable. The disruptions experienced since this virus came to town will have had a big impact on lots of aspects of your life, from work to exercise to cooking. You might feel stressed about your finances, anxious about going to the gym, or maybe you've slipped into midweek drinking and you're finding that hard to break. And if you're currently at home under restrictions, that can be stressful and boring too.

Maybe it's showing itself as a frustration at not being able to get motivated. Maybe it's the lack of physical activity compared to pre-virus times. Maybe you're craving physical touch. Maybe you're overloaded with news and information. Perhaps you're feeling worn out from too many Zoom video calls, or from trying to teach your kids at home while simultaneously trying to work or keep a toddler occupied. Or maybe it's this feeling of limbo — what happens next? What's the next stage?

Taking care of your wellbeing means prioritising better quality rest, so you can start to feel like you have a bit more energy. And that starts with the basics. If you sleep badly, don't eat well, and allow yourself to get into poor physical shape, you become far more likely to experience low moods. Daily chores can drain away what resources you have to cope and you can quickly start to feel down.

Keep an eye on what you eat: the stress of the pandemic can make you more likely to rebound into unhealthy eating habits. Lack of stimulation can do that too. Some people have likened their experience of lockdown to the longest long-haul flight ever: there's only so much TV you can watch, you feel trapped and resort to boredom eating, wishing it would all just be over, but the more you think this, the longer the journey seems to take. I can certainly relate to this.

Stress, tiredness and anxiety seem to have been the triggers that resulted in more than a quarter of people saying they had eaten less healthily during the early weeks of lockdown in the UK, according to a YouGov survey commissioned by the British Nutrition Foundation.[1] Boredom was the main reason people were eating more unhealthy food, but almost a third said that not being able to go to the supermarket had often made it difficult for them to eat well.

Exercise is good, but if you've been taking it easy for a while, make sure you build up gently so as to avoid risk of injury. In the YouGov survey, one third of those polled said they were spending more time sitting down than before lockdown, and 29% said that they were less active than usual. And it's easy to understand why. Personally, I tore my left calf muscle, not once but twice (same calf muscle, if you can believe that) in the period emerging out of lockdown in New Zealand. Throughout lockdown I'd been sitting at my desk a lot, as I worked hard to share advice and provide support on communication and wellbeing, so I was just not as active as I had been. I do wonder if this period of reduced activity made me much

1. https://www.nutrition.org.uk/attachments/article/1352/BNF HEW at home 2020 survey results Final_150620.pdf

more at risk of injury when I started moving around more again. That's a harsh and very painful personal lesson learned.

Getting a good night's sleep

With all the changes brought by this pandemic, many of us have found our sleep patterns interrupted. It's widely known that anxiety and a decline in mental wellbeing can negatively impact sleep.

Maybe you're waking up groggy, with that feeling of sleepiness still hanging around in your brain. You can't just wake up, switch on and then accelerate to 100 km/h; your brain needs a bit of time to warm up. Grogginess may be partly due to sleep hygiene issues — getting enough sleep, and enough good quality sleep — but it could also be due to a change in your routine.

If you're now working from home, in lockdown or have changed your morning routine, you may not be getting direct sunlight exposure early in the day, as you are no longer leaving the house early to get to work or going outside to shop or exercise. Outdoor light, particularly morning light, is one of the main biological signals to alertness, and lack of exposure makes you feel less alert throughout your whole day. Lack of direct sunlight exposure can cause your body clock to become misaligned, so that the body isn't ready to go to sleep when it's time to rest, resulting in less and lower quality sleep.

Some of us slipped into bad habits over lockdown, staying up late and watching Netflix in bed, or lying in bed while you clear your emails in the morning. In a survey from the American Academy of Sleep Medicine,[2] 88% reported that they had lost sleep due to binge watching, even though US adults ranked sleep as a top priority, second only to family. An average binge-watching session lasted three hours and eight minutes, with 52% of binge-watchers viewing three to four episodes in one sitting.

Aside from decreasing the quantity of sleep you can get, binge-watching affects the quality as well. All TVs, smartphones and tablets emit blue light. Research at Harvard Medical School[3] has shown that blue light artificially enhances attention, reaction times and mood — the opposite of what you want when trying to get a restorative night's rest.

Even the smallest amount of blue light inhibits the production of the sleep-regulating hormone melatonin. This, in turn, interrupts your circadian rhythm, the body's internal clock that regulates hormones, metabolism, and the sleep/wake cycle. It also delays the onset of quality REM rest, the most restorative component of the sleep cycle. None of this is good news.

Sacrificing sleep for entertainment can lead to frustration, worry and guilt particularly for Generation Z respondents.[4] While 24% of respondents admit feeling frustrated by missed bedtimes, nearly a third of Gen Z respondents feel frustrated full stop. These feelings can make the insufficient sleep problem worse, as negative thoughts about missing sleep might make it harder to fall asleep, especially when you try to make up for the lost time. And the Journal of Clinical Sleep Medicine found that binge-watchers reported more fatigue, more symptoms of insomnia, poorer sleep quality and greater alertness prior to going to sleep.

2. https://aasm.org/sleep-survey-binge-watching-results/
3. https://www.health.harvard.edu/staying-healthy/blue-light-has-a-dark-side
4. https://aasm.org/sleep-survey-binge-watching-results/

As for emails, waking up to a list of notifications can trigger troubling feelings. In a survey of nearly 2000 workers in the UK, the London-based Future Work Centre[5] found that email notifications are linked to higher feelings of anxiety. Do you really need that first thing in the morning?

Tristan Harris, Google's former Design Ethicist, has studied how technology exploits the mind's weakness to keep us checking our emails. When tech designers seek out and understand our blindspots, they can influence us without us even realising it, no matter how smart you are. Checking your emails first thing can derail your whole routine, because it frames your day around the list of things that you need to attend to as dictated by your tech devices, rather than what you choose to consciously prioritise.

In another analysis, at the University of British Columbia, researchers asked 124 students and professors to check their email frequently for one week.[6] The next week, they checked their email only three times per day and disabled all notifications. When time spent looking at email was restricted, the participants reported lower stress levels and higher feelings of positivity.

So instead of checking your email first thing in the morning, perhaps consider another activity that's more in line with your true needs. Coffee, anyone?

Another bad habit that could be affecting your sleep is checking the news too much, hitting refresh more often and getting caught up

5. Future Work Centre (2015). You've Got Mail Research Report. https://issuu.com/omnipsiconsulting/docs/fwc-youve-got-mail-research-report
6. Kushlev, K & Dunn, EW (2015). Checking email less frequently reduces stress. *Computers in Human Behavior*, 43:220–228. https://doi.org/10.1016/j.chb.2014.11.005

in an addictive news cycle. In the initial lockdown phase, research[7] showed that worry about Covid-19 was driving up news consumption, with 70% of Australians accessing news about it more than once per day. This consumption was driven by concern about the virus, with 78% of those who said they were worried about it, watching, reading and listening to news more often.

But among people who usually avoid the news, 71% were avoiding it more than usual too. This was largely driven by news fatigue. Women were more likely to avoid news about the coronavirus than men because they find it upsetting. Men were more likely to avoid it because they simply feel overwhelmed by the sheer volume of news.

While news about coronavirus provided people with an important shared topic of conversation, it also made people feel more anxious. According to the research, women were much more likely to feel an increase in anxiety because of coronavirus news (59%) than men (44%), and younger people found the news coverage more anxiety-inducing than older people, particularly Gen Y (people born 1981–1996). This may seem odd given that older people are more likely to suffer serious health effects, but job losses, isolation from friends, school closures and uncertainty about the future all impact younger people.

All of this resulted in a push-and-pull dynamic regarding the news, with anxiety driving people to check news more often, while simultaneously pulling us to avoid further news information. It's tiring to try to manage this dynamic all the time.

7. COVID-19: Australian news and misinformation (2020) by Sora Park, Caroline Fisher, Jee Young Lee and Kieran McGuinness, News & Media Research Centre, University of Canberra.

Anxiety doesn't help either. Even if we are just experiencing low-grade, background-level anxiety rather than acute bouts, it's likely to affect the duration and quality of your sleep. And this can add up over a period of time. Your sleep may well have been affected for a while before you start to actually feel tired, although it's likely that your cognitive performance — how quickly you're able to solve problems and be mentally agile — has also been affected for a while, but you just haven't noticed it.

So what can you do?

1. **Limit your news intake.** Try to limit yourself to checking the news once or at the most twice a day. Find out what you need to know and then get out of there. That way you won't miss any important announcements or updates, but you also help to manage any anxiety and overwhelm you might be experiencing too. And do not do your infrequent news check-in just before bedtime. Give yourself a good buffer of at least a couple of hours between checking the news and the time when you want to be calm and ready to sleep.
2. **Limit your time social media.** Social media is great for connecting but it can also be tempting to spend too long on it, making yourself ever more anxious.
3. **Take in the sun.** Try to get 30–90 minutes of direct sunlight exposure before 12 noon. Go for a walk, or sit or do your work near a window. Even if it's cloudy outside, the light is still enough to do its thing with your body clock.
4. **Exercise.** Movement and activity influence our quality of sleep, and even a short online workout will help tire you out.
5. **Keep the bedroom for sleeping.** Create clear boundaries for working, relaxing and socialising at home and keep the bedroom separate.
6. **Work with your chronotype.** If you know that you're a morning person or a night person, then it's best to work with

your natural setting, rather than against it.

7. **Routine.** Trying to stick to a structure every day will help with not only sleep but mental health too. Make it a rule that you go to bed (and to sleep) at the same time each evening. The sleep you get before midnight seems to be better value than the sleep your get after midnight, so try to get to bed earlier.

8. **Try not to nap.** This can break down your rhythm of regular bedtimes and waking times.

Video calls and screen time

Another factor that could be contributing to your fatigue is video calls. Whether you're working from home, managing your child's schoolwork, or just trying to stay in touch with friends and relatives who live far away, many of us are doing a lot of video calls these days.

What is it about Zoom, Teams and other video calls that make us feel so tired? For starters, you're probably doing a lot more than you usually would. If you're working from home and don't have to travel between meetings, it's so tempting to pop another Zoom call into that slot, because it looks like you have more available time now.

But humans tend to crave variety and when so many aspects of our lives come together in one medium, that contributes to a feeling of exhaustion. On a video call you typically see yourself as well as the other callers and that makes us more self-aware, and perhaps self-conscious too. It's as if you're now on stage, all the time. Then there are the inevitable tech glitches. When there's a silence in the dialogue, you find yourself wondering whether they didn't like what you said or the screen has frozen.

If you're in lockdown, you could easily find yourself on video calls for most of the waking hours in your day. You're also probably not getting up and moving around as much as you normally would pre-Covid-19 times, so it can feel like an extended staring competition with a roomful of strangers.

So what can you do to ease the exhaustion caused by video calls?

1. Cut back on the number of Zoom or video call meetings, and spread them across the day — maybe two or three calls in the morning and again in the afternoon. Max out there and make sure you have at least 10 minutes between meetings so you can move around. This might mean aiming to wrap up a meeting after 50 minutes so you can use the remaining 10 minutes in the hour to go for a quick walk — or just do something else before the next call!

2. If you don't need to meet on video, try picking up the phone. This gives your brain a break, because you're not having to do the visual interpretive work of trying to match the body language to what is being said.

3. Use a background. Video calls can feel like you're opening up your home for others to view and, for some of us, that can trigger social comparison worries. If your kids are using Zoom, then they might prefer not to have people prying around at stuff behind them either. On Zoom, you can change the settings so that instead of seeing your room behind you, the other party sees a backdrop image.

4. Use speaker view. That way, the person speaking is maximised on screen while everyone else is minimised. This means you don't need to have the self-consciousness of always monitoring yourself, and you can turn down that feeling of being stared at by a roomful of strangers.

5. Take breaks. If you're also socialising using video chat, ask yourself how much of one communication channel can you deal with in your life right now? Pick up the phone or send a message and add some variety to the way you communicate.

While we're thinking about video calls, it's worth considering what your screen time looks like now, compared to what you were doing before Covid-19. How were you doing your work, or spending your time before the virus? Has it changed much? How long and how often are you on the screen, and what are you actually doing? Are you working, absorbing information, passively scrolling and looking at pictures, or are you commenting and posting?

It helps to break down screen time a bit, because not all screen time is the same. If I'm creating videos, or editing in YouTube Studio, or doing my research, then for me that also counts as creative time. If I'm checking Twitter, Facebook and news sites, as well as catching up on email, then I treat that time differently.

Once you've got a good idea of how much and how you are using screens, consider how you feel about your current screen use. Does it need to stay the way it is now? What could you be doing with your time instead that you might be missing out on?

Don't beat yourself up, but take it as an opportunity to glean some insight into habits that might stick. Choose to be a bit more intentional — decide whether you're fine with it carrying on like this for a while, or whether you might want to make a shift towards a different pattern of screen use.

Fatigue

Even if you are getting enough sleep, there's another factor that might be making you feel more tired than usual. If you're living under shifting restrictions or in lockdown, you may notice that you feel tired, exhausted and somehow drained. It's not lack of sleep, it's just that things feel somehow heavy. It's a worrying time.

In our pre-Covid days we would make dozens of low-impact decisions every day and not think twice about them. *Go for a coffee in the usual place before I get to work — sure! Head over to see Grandpa up the coast this weekend — let's make it a surprise! He'll be so happy to see us.*

Now these low-impact decisions have become moral dilemmas to wrestle with. Whether it's deciding to get together in a group on the weekend, take public transport, shake someone's hand or even head to the supermarket, we have to think through the potential implications of everyday actions and decisions in a way we've never had to before, because of how they could affect others.

As much as we'd like to believe that we're all lone wolves who can fend for ourselves and prioritise our own best interests, in reality that's never how it worked. It's a fiction to think that we're not already deeply connected to one another — we always have been, it's just that the consequences now have been ratcheted up in a different way. Even our most simple actions and decisions can now have moral consequences that impact someone else's life and health very significantly.

This tiredness and weight is called moral fatigue and it's exhausting. It's also sneaky — you experience it without recognising the added burden you're carrying. There seems to be more at stake in terms of these everyday decisions, both for ourselves, our loved ones and others around us; we're just not used to having to consider severe possible consequences resulting from normal everyday errands and tasks.

As exhausting as moral fatigue can be, we're experiencing it because we're taking the time to reflect more on how our decisions and actions may affect other people. The added strain and effort, on the one hand, is unpleasant and complicates our lives. But on the other hand, it's potentially a very good thing, because the alternative is to live the usual oblivious life where we don't recognise our interdependence.

What can you do? Well, talking with supportive friends and family can be really helpful in terms of processing feelings, normalising fears and doubts, and talking through decision-making. But break it up and take things one day at a time. Anxiety has a way of making everything feel super-urgent. It convinces us that things must happen right now, when that's simply not the case.

Relieving muscle stress

When you feel anxious, you might notice strain or tension in your muscles and this can make your anxiety more difficult to manage in the moment. By relieving the muscle stress, you can begin to reduce your anxiety levels. Here's how to do it:

Sit in a quiet and comfortable place.

Close your eyes and focus on your breathing.

Breathe slowly in through your nose and out of your mouth.

Use your hand to make a tight fist. Squeeze your fist tightly. Hold your squeezed fist for a few seconds. Notice all the tension you feel in your hand.

Slowly open your fingers and be aware of how you feel. You may notice a feeling of tension leaving your hand. Eventually, your hand will feel lighter and more relaxed.

Continue tensing and then releasing various muscle groups in your body, from your hands, legs, shoulders, or feet. You may want to work your way up and down your body, tensing various muscle groups. Avoid tensing the muscles in any area of your body where you're injured or in pain, as that might aggravate your injury.

Keep practising this technique and you'll start to notice a difference. You can feel the tension and you can just let it go.

Alcohol and Covid-19

Another factor that can impact on your energy and fatigue is alcohol. During those long, isolated days at home, whether in lockdown or simply socially isolated, many people found their drinking patterns were altered.

Some people who don't usually drink carried on quite happily like that, while others began drinking again after a period of abstinence. Some cut down because drinking is a person-to-person social thing, while others found a new way to socially drink, hosting virtual parties over video conference apps. Some drank because they were bored, to mark the end of a long week, or celebrate just getting through another school day.

Perhaps you, like many others around the world, picked up a lockdown habit of having an alcoholic drink to mark the end of another long and isolated day. If you did, you're not alone. The worst pandemic in 100 years has driven many people to drink. A breathalyser app in the United States, which logs average blood alcohol among its users, showed a spike in several US cities after they passed stay-at-home orders.[8] Alcoholic drink sales shot up around the world, even being labelled as an essential item to make sure that supply chains were maintained and wine, beer, cider and spirits could still make it through the shops to your home.

If your drinking habits have changed, it's important to get clear on your reason for drinking. Perhaps you are drinking to take the edge off your anxiety, or your boredom, or to connect with others over video calls on a Friday night. We know that drinking can increase when people go through stressful conditions. Addiction services here in New Zealand reported a rise in drinking, cannabis use and online gambling over the lockdown period.[9]

8. https://www.bactrack.com/pages/coronavirus-covid-19-causing-dramatic-shift-alcohol-drinking-habits-americans-lockdown
9. https://www.drugfoundation.org.nz/assets/uploads/2020-uploads/

Having a beer at the end of a hard day isn't by itself a bad thing. The important thing is to consider how much your overall consumption has increased, how long you plan to continue at that level and whether there is something else you could be doing instead.

One of the problems is that people vastly underestimate how much they drink. While it may not constitute 'binge drinking' to consume two drinks a night, that amount does increase our risk of getting sick, in a number of different ways. People who are having more than a glass of wine (and not one of those big ones) are actually increasing their risk of severe disease and in a way we can't quantify it until it gets to be too much, and then you become ill.

Alcohol changes levels of serotonin and other neurotransmitters in the brain, which can worsen anxiety. In fact, you may feel more anxious after the alcohol wears off. Alcohol-induced anxiety can actually last for several hours or even for an entire day after drinking. Plus drinking more heavily might also make us a bit less careful or responsible about things like hand washing and physical distancing.

No matter what your reason for drinking, it's important to remember that the more you drink, the more you're likely to drink. And the risk is that as we increase our drinking, we run the risk of increasing out set-point, or what we now think is a normal level of drinking. That one glass can turn to two glasses almost every night. And perhaps more. And this might then normalise a habit that we find hard to break, especially as the uncertainty and restrictions could continue for some time.

So yes, alcohol can feel good in the short term — it's a culturally

Covid-19-resources/Pulse-survey-of-addiction-services-and-people-who-use-drugs-during-alert-level-4.pdf acceptable way to unwind and relax in many places and societies in the world. It's one of those things that many people just do. But it's not very sustainable, because every time you go to have another drink, you get a little less benefit from the buzz. Some people find that 'performative boozing', pouring a drink at 5.30pm to try to mark the evening had started, actually doesn't work for them in the end. And once they've had a few days off, people often find they like how they feel and carry on not drinking — not necessarily forever, but at least for a time.

Have a think about what patterns you may have grown accustomed to over the lockdown period, and if this is something you want to continue with. Perhaps drink-free days are already a regular part of your life? If not, perhaps introducing some of these into your week might be a good starting point.

These are not hard and fast rules, where if you happen to drink two glasses of wine you're somehow now a bad person. People are struggling right now, and it's not wrong to seek ways to cope. But it's good to diversify the ways of coping that you have in your toolbox.

CHAPTER 10

Mastering your brake

Stop for a moment and consider how you are feeling at the moment. How is your mood generally? Are you finding yourself up and down? Or maybe you're feeling pretty low, pretty much all of the time?

Whatever you're feeling, recognise that it's normal to feel battered about a bit. This has been a prolonged period of adjustment and then readjustment, with more uncertainty yet to come. You'd almost be superhuman if you weren't feeling the mental strain by now.

The question is, how are you dealing with that mental strain?

Everyone responds differently to a crisis. By now it's inevitable that you've experienced or witnessed some coping strategies — both yours and someone else's — that could be less than ideal.

So what is coping anyway? Coping is all about responding effectively to problems and challenges. When you cope well, you're responding to a threat in a way that tries to minimise its damaging impact.

But we can choose many different strategies in order to cope and they tend to fall into one of two different categories: problem-focused and emotion-focused strategies.

Problem-focused strategies are all about actively engaging with the outside world in order to deal with the threat. This might mean making plans, getting more information, or confronting the threat or adversary head-on. Emotion-focused coping is instead directed inwards. It's all about attempting to change how we respond emotionally to stressful events, rather than trying to do something about the event itself.

Effective emotion-focused strategies might include meditation, humour and trying to see the silver lining in bad events. Less effective emotion-focused strategies might include denial, distraction, and substance use. Although they might work in the short term, they don't address the actual cause of the event, or prevent its longer-term effects.

Neither problem-solving nor emotion-focused coping strategies are intrinsically more or less effective than the other. Both can be effective for different kinds of challenges. In some contexts in this pandemic, problem-focused coping such as washing your hands, wearing a mask and socially distancing are going to be advised and work well for you. But if you're overwhelmed by anxiety, then maybe we need to focus on being able to manage that inwardly first.

Problem-focused strategies tend to work best when we can control the problem. But when we have an insurmountable or immovable problem, it can be better to adjust our response to emotion-focused strategies rather than banging our heads against a problem where we have little control.

Hopefully, you can see why this pandemic has been so tricky. As our understanding of the virus has changed, we have been able to develop more sophisticated ways of trying to control the problem. But these ways of controlling the virus spread brings up anxiety, frustration, anger, despondency and a whole host of other emotions for people that can feel overwhelming. People find it difficult to focus on problem-solving strategies until they can deal with those emotions first. To a certain extent, it's a bit of a chicken and egg situation unless we learn how to carefully navigate this.

The first step is to understand how we can get conscious control over our threat management system that tends to determine our first coping response, which is all about keeping us alive. It's only once we can consciously control what coping strategy we will use that we can get better control over ourselves and how we can meet the challenges ahead.

This chapter is all about mastering the brake, so that our primal survival system doesn't get to call all the shots. Because although it might keep you alive, it doesn't really help you to pay attention to an ever-changing threat, or adapt to truly start living again, in spite of the threat.

So how does this unfold in real terms? As you sit back and watch the painful consequences of a global pandemic unfold on the news, fear switches off your rational brain, and your threat brain swings into action, screaming at you to quit focusing on normal everyday tasks (like work) and deal with the basics: EAT FOOD. PLAY DEAD. FIGHT ANYONE WHO MESSES WITH YOU.

Some of these responses aren't necessarily bad. If you're experiencing acute anxiety, watching a video of a dog pushing around another dog in a shopping trolley is probably a great way to calm down. Or at least it's one of them.

But it's also entirely possible to indulge in too much 'self-care'. When you find yourself unhealthily bingeing on things that comfort you — whether it's food, TV, sleep, or video games — you're being avoidant. In the long term, this can lead to dissociation, which is bad for your brain and body.

Dissociation means being disconnected from the present moment.

It is a subconscious way of coping and avoiding a traumatic situation or negative thoughts. That can be helpful in a moment of acute stress, because it helps you do what you need to do to help yourself and others. When your child is injured and screaming in pain, many parents find instead of collapsing in a bundle of tears and shock, they can stay calm and do what is needed to treat the injury. That's disassociation operating as a protective mechanism and helping you to get through that moment.

So dissociation works to get you through the short term, but if it's something you find yourself doing all the time, dissociation can shut you off from the world, causing you to feel disconnected and helpless. It can make it hard to feel like you can bear others' pain, which in turn can disempower you from doing good. And all of that can make your recovery from this trauma harder once things normalise.

So what can you do to feel more like your old self? It's vital to note that punishing yourself — telling yourself you're a slob who just needs to push through it all — won't work. Shame and guilt actually cause an increase in stress hormones in your body, which can trigger your anxious brain even more.

In our society, we're so often taught that speed and efficacy are better. But to get your logical brain back online, you actually need the opposite: mindfulness, calmness, and silence. And if you want to talk long-term productivity, spending 30 minutes on effective mindfulness techniques saves a lot more time than hours of mindless scrolling, struggling to focus on that thing you are supposed to be getting done.

Let's talk about disappointment

By now it's inevitable that you've experienced some

disappointments as a result of this virus. When significant events happen in our lives, we participate in rituals to commemorate, to come together, and to help us to move on. Those rituals may not be available to us right now, or at least not in the same way. Weddings have been postponed, graduations are missed; school camps that have been long planned for are cancelled and school itself might be difficult to attend for months on end. All this takes a cumulative toll.

It's not surprising that you might feel disappointed from time to time, when you think about all the things you wish you could do but can't right now. When you get disappointed, it can hurt. Sometimes a bit. Sometimes a lot. It can drag you down into a negative funk for days or even weeks.

If you learn how to deal with that disappointment in a healthier and more helpful way, then it can be a lot less scary and painful, and it won't stick around as long.

Here's how:

1. Recognise that disappointment is a normal part of life

Remind yourself that disappointment will happen if you go outside of your comfort zone — and in these times, pretty much everyone is operating outside their comfort zone for at least part of the time. Experiencing setbacks and feeling disappointed is a natural part of living your life. Disappointment hurts and it's okay to acknowledge that. Just remember to remind yourself that you can live with it.

2. Take a wider perspective

One of the most powerful ways to deal with your disappointment is by letting it out into the light. By talking the situation over with a close friend or loved one, you can begin to see the situation from another perspective.

Taking a healthier and broader perspective is a vital step in processing your disappointment and moving forward. The key is being open to hearing that fresh perspective, rather than seeking an opportunity to nurture and feed your disappointment (something we are all capable of when left to our own devices).

Ask your loved one not to simply agree with you, but to present another perspective on the situation. Together, you can come up with the start of an action plan for how you will move forward. This conversation will help you ground yourself and resist the temptation to create a mountain out of a molehill.

3. Quit the comparison trap

'Comparison is the thief of joy', according to Theodore Roosevelt. If you compare what you can do now to what you could do before, or you compare your life to other people's lives, or life in other cities or countries, then you can easily start to feel depressed and bad about yourself and your efforts.

There will always be people doing things differently to you and sharing only their best selves on social media. Comparison is a destructive trap and you don't have to buy into it. Notice when you are comparing, and focus on your own progress — measure where you are now compared to last week, last month or last year and appreciate what you have achieved. That might not look like a lot, but remember that these are extraordinary times. Social media is a curated garden. You get to see what people want you to see, not their clothes strewn all over the bedroom floor, mixed in with five-day-old pizza boxes.

4. Shift your focus from what you lack to what you have

Practising gratitude helps us refocus on what we have instead of what we lack. Tapping into gratitude can help you to put things into perspective and prevent a disappointment from overwhelming you and derailing your whole day or week.

The gratitude jars

Take two jars. Label one 'Gratitude' and the other 'Deferred Wishes'.

Each day, take a slip of paper and write down a list of things you are grateful for. This could be anything, including — or perhaps especially — the basics many of us take for granted, like a roof over your head and clean water, a hot cup of tea, a cool breeze or the smile of a loved one. Add the date and put the slip into the Gratitude jar. If you like, you can invite everyone in the household to contribute.

Practising gratitude may feel a bit forced and contrived at first, but this mental state grows stronger with use.

The Deferred Wishes jar is for all the things you wish that you could do, that are simply not possible right now. Don't give up those wishes, just park them in this jar for now. That overseas dream trip might have to wait for a bit longer, but you can also add simple things like meeting your best mate for a decent coffee or attending a concert, free of worry about the virus. Write them all down and look forward to being able to do them someday soon.

When you decide to open the jars in a few weeks or months, it will be interesting to reflect on what you've written down.

The dates will help you make sense of how your gratitudes and wishes have changed over time. What was important to you a few months ago may not feel so important now. You might also see different patterns — some members of the family might be more grateful for some things than others.

The Deferred Wishes jar will be like a treasure trove of things to do when 'normal' life returns someday soon. Hold on to it. The virus won't last forever.

Fear about the future

Alongside those actual disappointments, there's more uncertainty to deal with, like what will happen to your child's school, college or university next term? What about that trip you've got planned? Will that wedding go ahead? What happens when the baby is born, or a loved one passes away? When will you get to see overseas family again? Will the virus resurge? Will we face lockdown and restrictions again? And what about your finances?

When we start looking too far into the future, we might feel our anxiety levels starting to rise. Some of this anxiety comes from feeling out of control, like there's nothing we can do about all these things that are important for your daily life. You can't even make reliable plans or book a holiday.

All this fear and anxiety about the future can rev us up into fight or flight mode. We may feel in our bodies a shortness of breath, or a racing heart. It's like the anxiety accelerator in our bodies has been pushed flat to the floor and we are doing doughnuts in the car park.

This revved up anxiety can be a problem, especially at times when we're asked to stay at home or self-isolate. We don't want to be fighting with loved ones or lashing out online and it won't always be possible to get the physical space you need.

So how can you deal with anxiety? Ignoring the feelings or squashing them down won't make them go away, so try making space for them instead.

Slow belly-breathing

When you feel your anxiety revving up, simply hit the brakes with some slow belly-breathing.

Set a timer for 60 seconds and breathe in through your nose and out through your mouth, counting each breath. Take good full breaths — not too fast and not too slow. Just breathe normally, inflating and deflating your belly in each breath. You can close your eyes, or look down at the floor.

Put this book down now and give it a go.

How many breaths did you manage in 60 seconds? There is no right answer, but once you know how many breaths you take in 60 seconds, you won't even need a timer. You can use this technique any time you feel like you need to slow down a bit, or want to feel a bit less shaky and anxious.

The beauty of this is that it only takes 60 seconds to change what is happening in your body and shift from revving up to slowing down.

Try it again right now and see what happens.

Feels good, right?

Dealing with frustration

Frustration, irritation with yourself and others, and distress are common experiences when we are under chronic stress and it feels like there is no way out. When your stress hormones are continually pumping because your threat system is active, it's hard to see things as they are.

Frustration can impact your life in many different ways. You may feel irritable, get snappy with loved ones, or have weird dreams or nightmares. Some research suggests that when people experience frustration in the day, they tend to have more frightening dreams at night. It's as if the mind is trying to process and make sense of experiences we find psychologically distressing when we are awake. Throw in disturbed sleep, lack of stimulation and reduced social contact, and you can see that it's easy to end up in quite a downward loop.

When that happens, it's natural that you would start to seek some relief from the frustration. You might start looking for ways around some of the restrictions, just so you can get some sense of normality and control. You start thinking that maybe it doesn't matter so much if you nip out without your mask, or have 12 people in the room when the current guidelines say no more than 10. (It does matter. Please don't.)

Bear in mind that men and women tend to express anger and frustration differently. Both feel anger and frustration, yet men tend to accept and embrace the emotions, using them to their advantage. In contrast, women tend to view anger and frustration as counterproductive and often camouflage these emotions due to social expectations of behaviour. One study found that in general, when asked to hold their emotions in, men felt ineffective, while women did not feel so constricted.

Here are four tips to help you deal with your frustration so you can soothe yourself, and keep yourself and others safe.

1. Take some deep breaths. It's likely that the frustration you're feeling has caused you to hold your breath or breathe shallowly. This means your body is oxygen-depleted and it's hard to think clearly. When you take a few deep breaths, your pent-up emotions will start to ease and you can restore a sense of calm. Deep breathing can also help slow your heartbeat and lower your blood pressure, reducing the negative effects of frustration and irritation.

2. Remove the 'noise' and simplify. When you're finding things difficult, figure out what's absolutely necessary and remove everything else. If you just need to stay in your pyjamas all day and watch TV with the kids, then do it. Get yourself into a better place, and start again when you can.

3. Keep track of your wins. When a difficult situation is dragging on, it's easy to lose track of what is going well. Keep a win log, update it daily and be sure to review it weekly. When you have a moment of happiness, a great game with your kids, or a good chat with a friend or loved one, write it down. When you review your win log at the end of the week, you may be surprised by how much you have done and how many great things happened.

4. Remind yourself that this will pass. Frustration shouldn't be an ongoing experience. Like the weather, it's bound to change. By recognising that emotions are generally fleeting, you rob them of their power and hold on you. Try to envision yourself in a happier place and remember that things that have frustrated you in the past generally didn't last that long. Either you found ways to get past it, or the things that frustrated you often did not have a lasting impact.

Shaking off the doom and gloom

So what if you find yourself dwelling on doom and gloom? You start off with a negative thought and your brain spirals further and further down, leaving you anxious, glum and depressed.

This is a normal response to a stressful situation, because the human brain is genetically wired to detect negative information or threats, faster than positive information or opportunities. Our prehistoric ancestors were acutely aware that if they missed an opportunity, there would likely be another one coming. But if they missed a threat, they might not live to see either another threat or an opportunity. Because, well, you might be dead.

Neuroscientists call this automatic habit of the brain 'negativity bias'. It's useful because it helps us to be acutely aware of the negative so we live to see another day. The evidence of this lies in our amygdala and reptilian brain, which is our 'search and destroy or get the hell out of the way!' system.

In modern times, however, this habit of the brain leaves us reacting to a stroppy email or difficult conversation as if our life were in danger. It activates a cascade of stress hormones and leaves us fixated on potential threats, unable to see the bigger picture.

Unfortunately, we are wired to obsess over the negative. The human brain is like Velcro for negative experiences — they stick around and our brain makes us notice them. And it's like Teflon for positive experiences — telling us to pay no attention as another opportunity will come along.

So how can we shift our negativity bias so that we avoid wallowing in doom and gloom?

The key thing to understand is that brain habits are like plastic: strong enough to resist the occasional push but malleable enough to change in response to repeated effort with a technique known as Notice-Shift-Rewire. Here's how to do it:

Notice-Shift-Rewire

1. Notice your brain's negativity bias. It's not your fault — it was built this way, but bring some awareness to this ordinary habit of your mind. Catch yourself when you slip into self-doubt, rumination, anxiety, and fear. Notice when your mind starts spinning out worst-case scenarios about how it's all going to come crashing apart.

2. Shift to noticing a positive experience. Noticing opens the space for connecting new neural pathways and shifting allows you to flood this space with a more productive focus of attention. A few seconds of gratitude is the most efficient way to do this, so think of one thing you're grateful for right now. Your health. Your family. Your talents and strengths.

3. Rewire by Savouring. This is where the work of rewiring starts to happen. Take 15 seconds to stay with this new grateful mindset so you can encode it deep into the fabric of your mind. This is where we transform our ordinary habit of overlooking the positive and shift the brain's response to all the good in life.

In this way we can switch the roles of our Velcro and Teflon. We're flipping our evolved wiring on its head by taking a few seconds to imprint stronger memories about good things happening in life.

CHAPTER 11

Long-term stress

Existential anxiety

In 1844, Danish philosopher Søren Kierkegaard wrote: 'Whoever has learnt to be anxious in the right way, has learnt the ultimate.'

I'm no Kierkegaard, but I think he may have been on to something. The anxiety we may be experiencing in these coronavirus times might be something that feels different, deeper, and beyond perhaps your usual fear or anxiety about day-to-day troubles. This feels more existential.

Existential usually means feelings of unease about meaning, choice, and freedom in life. Whatever you call it, the main concerns are the same: the idea is that life is inherently pointless, that our existence has no meaning because there are limits or boundaries on it, and that we all must die someday.

That may sound pretty bleak, but it's not an uncommon experience. It's just that we don't talk about it very much, and when we do experience it, we feel like we might be alone in our experience, so we keep it covered up.

An existential crisis often occurs after major life events, such as career or job change, death of a loved one, diagnosis of a serious or life-threatening illness, a significant birthday, experiencing a tragic or traumatic experience, having children, divorce or even marriage.

For existentialists, an existential crisis is considered to be a journey, a necessary experience and a complex phenomenon. It comes from an awareness of your own freedoms and how life will end for you one day. That journey may reveal to us that where there was structure and familiarity, now there is mystery, unfamiliarity, a sense of discomfort and a feeling like somehow, things don't fit so well any more.

Where there was certainty, there is now uncertainty and unpredictability, meaning that we need to find our way again, in a place and time that feels unfamiliar to us. What served us well as navigation points in our lives perhaps don't serve us well any more, and we find ourselves wondering what happens now, without much in the way of a script to help us.

Strangely enough, this sense of existential anxiety could have become worse with the easing of restrictions and re-entry into some form of regular life. During lockdown, the structures provided by the government gave us some sense of certainty, at least in New Zealand and phrases like the 'team of five million' helped people band together. Research shows that connecting, especially through collective action, can mitigate the impact of disasters on our mental health and sense of agency.

Once restrictions were eased, New Zealand was almost an outlier on the world stage. Our geographic remoteness coupled with border restrictions that make it logistically hard to get here (and hard to leave too) can contribute to a sense of isolation and collective loneliness. It can lead us to question what meaning there was in this collective action if we are left with uncertainty now.

In many places in the world, you may be uncertain about the coronavirus itself — how it is tracking, whether it will continue to spread and whether you yourself or your loved ones may fall ill with it, or worse.

But what if you didn't have to solve this anxiety? Existentialists would argue that anxiety is an inevitable part of life that everyone will experience, so it isn't something that we aim to eliminate, but it might be something we need to learn to live with instead.

Around the world, many people have found that the Covid-19 crisis has helped them realise what is truly important in their lives. The basics: like health, relationships, a safe and warm place you can call home, dignity, freedom from persecution and discrimination. Being able to feed yourself and pay the bills.

In this way, an existential crisis might move you towards greater authenticity, which may also bring anxiety as you struggle for meaning. Now that the familiarity of your life has been stripped bare, what is your life really about? You might have thoughts about the fleetingness of your existence and how you are living it. When you stop taking for granted that you will wake up each day alive, you might experience anxiety, but at the same time deeper meaning too. These are actually two sides of the same coin.

Because of this, each of us must find a way to 'live with' this anxiety rather than try to eliminate it. Experiencing an existential crisis can also be positive; it can guide you to question your purpose in life and help provide direction.

So how can you turn an existential crisis into a positive experience for you or someone you love?

1. **Write it down.** Can you let this existential anxiety motivate you and guide you towards a more authentic life? What can this anxiety teach you about your relatedness to the world? Pull out a notebook and jot down your thoughts on these questions. It's in the answers to these questions that you may find how to cope with an existential crisis.
2. **Seek support.** Talking with loved ones about your existential

anxiety can help you gain a different life perspective and remind you of the positive impact you've had on their lives. Ask them to help you identify your most positive and admirable qualities. If you feel like that might be difficult for you, then you can find a trusted and qualified mental health professional instead and perhaps reflect with them on what's troubling you.

3. **Meditation.** Meditation can help you to reduce negative thoughts and help prevent anxiety and obsessive worry linked to an existential crisis. Meditation is a good way to practise sitting with uncomfortable thoughts, since learning to acknowledge these thoughts and then let them go helps increase your sense of control over them. One of the more common forms is mindfulness meditation and while it's not a universal panacea, it does seem to be particularly beneficial for people who tend to fall prey to obsessive ruminations and constantly turning over worries in their minds. Check out the mindful breathing exercise in chapter 2.

Meditation can be beneficial, but more recent research has found that it's not helpful for everyone. If you want to try meditating, a good place to start is the free guided meditations hosted at the UCLA Mindful Awareness Research Center.[1]

There is no specific treatment for dealing with existential anxiety, but there are treatments that can be helpful. For example, cognitive behavioural therapy (CBT) and medication can help to address symptoms of anxiety, depression, and other mental health issues that may accompany existential anxiety, including thoughts of suicide.

1. https://www.uclahealth.org/marc/mindful-meditations

In the end, the process of learning to live with this existential anxiety should possibly be framed as adaptation rather than recovery. Adaptation means being able to constantly move as conditions change, rather than trying to recover to some imaginary fixed point which may or may never happen. Recovery implies that this will all be over at some fixed point in time and we can somehow make our way back to where we were before, in terms of our lifestyles, our goals and dreams, as well as broader aspects such as the economy and what it was focused on.

It's clear that a lot of things will change as a result of this pandemic. It is also clear that the recovery will not be marked by a discrete event. More likely it will be a much messier adaptation. First, we must await the delivery of effective vaccines that have been proven to be both effective and safe. We will have to determine who gets priority access and iron out any inequities of access both between and within countries, as well as the inevitable ethical dilemmas that will arise, as well as both vaccine hesitancy and the deliberate spread of misinformation. From my work as Vaccine Policy Coordinator for the UK government during the H1N1 (swine flu) epidemic of 2009–10, I know that all of this takes time and is a vigorously contested space, not always fought on facts.

Meanwhile, the virus will continue to travel across the world, and within communities, exploiting any gaps in protection measures. We don't yet know how this will play out, but we can be certain of the uncertainty the pandemic will continue to create, and of our need to live with and adapt to it safely, while taking measures to protect both health and livelihoods.

Silver linings

Of all the things that you've had to change due to Covid-19, there's no doubt a few you'd be happy to give up right away. But what have you learned about yourself that you want to carry forward into your life? How have restrictions and lockdowns moved you towards greater authenticity and understanding of what's important to you?

Some people have realised that they weren't spending enough time with their children, and they're thinking about how that might change for them in the future. Some people have discovered that they love or hate working from home. Either way, it's going to change how they do things in the future. And some people have a newfound appreciation for the takeaway meal, as they don't ever want to cook all the time again.

These five questions will help you think about what you have liked or valued about this time, and what you want to take with you as we journey forwards. Write as much or as little as you want.

1. Write about someone or something that has been very important to you during your experience of living through this time of Covid-19.
2. Write about three things you are grateful for over this time, and why.
3. Make a list of 10 things you wish you knew before we embarked on this Covid-19 journey.
4. Write about one thing that you did over the past few weeks that you are proud of.
5. Write about 10 things you'd say yes to and 10 things you'd say no to, if you had to do this all over again.

Talk about your findings with family and friends. When you

identify the blessings, you can start to make subtle changes so that you live more in alignment with what's truly important for you. It will also help you prepare for the future, especially if you end up facing restrictions again.

The long-term impacts

So does this existential anxiety mean we are going to need a huge mental health programme to help people cope with the impacts of coronavirus on individual lives and society? Or do we need something else instead?

Although Covid-19 is a very different kind of crisis compared to those that many places in the world have faced recently, what we already know about getting through a crisis is relevant and helpful here. We also need to think about what drives common mental health issues outside of Covid-19 times, in order to figure out how best to help ourselves and each other.

When we talk about disasters or a crisis, we often focus on the disruption and stress caused by the event itself — the tornado, the hurricane, the earthquake. In the case of Covid-19, we might think of the health impact of the virus on people and communities as the immediate shock.

In the immediate aftermath of a disaster, we know that survivors can experience a range of psychosocial symptoms such as stress, grief, depression and anxiety. Studies show that while the majority experience passing distress, most people, given the appropriate resources and support, return to a relatively stable pattern of healthy functioning in time. That's not to say that they won't feel anxious or sad from time to time, but it does mean that these are common responses that tend to be managed reasonably well when people have access to the social support they need and are getting their basic needs met.

There is clearly a need to offer mental health support for many of those affected by Covid-19, including patients who have had really rough experiences, and possible post-traumatic stress issues for those who have been working hard helping others in very busy or trying circumstances.

For others who are struggling and feel like they don't have the personal resources to cope effectively, there is certainly a place for mental health services and prescribed medication, where appropriate. But rather than just treating the symptoms, it's helpful to look at the causes and do something about those too. And those causes have been around long before coronavirus times.

Loneliness is already a major mental health challenge in our increasingly individualistic society. We know that how connected we are with each other determines how we develop a shared sense of purpose and meaning as individuals, families and communities. Research has shown that even simply knowing you can borrow $100 in a time of need helps to bolster the sense that we are not alone and strengthens our wellbeing.

For some people, loneliness has increased with restrictions, particularly in some places where these have gone on and on. Evidence suggests that physical distancing measures can also increase mental distress. Some people have felt scared, angry, lonely, stressed, bored or frustrated with the constraints of movement restrictions, being confined to 'bubbles' at home, and not being able to come into contact with people other than those who share your living space.

But loneliness isn't just about isolation, and feeling lonely is not the same as being alone. Loneliness is a feeling of disconnection. It's the sense that no one around you really understands you and that you don't have the kind of meaningful connections you would like. You can feel lonely in a crowd, just as you can feel perfectly happy, even relieved, to spend some time alone. Loneliness is a factor because it's that feeling of disconnection — and we know that a good level of social support and connection is a protective factor when going through a crisis.

In these cases, it doesn't make sense to treat the anxiety alone. Addressing the lack of social support and finding ways to build a sense of connection will go a long way towards addressing loneliness and easing the anxiety.

Secondary stressors

Just as important as the crisis itself — perhaps more important over the long term — are secondary stressors. These are knock-on effects of the initial event that create emotional strain among survivors, making it more difficult to get back to 'normal'. Things like financial strain, relationship difficulties, education disruptions, delayed insurance claim resolution, inability to travel, and job insecurity or loss.

While physical distancing and restrictions on movement were necessary to protect health and wellbeing, adopting these public health measures may result in secondary stress for mental wellbeing. People might also experience a loss of agency and control, as restrictions shape their lives in ways that are starkly different to pre-Covid times.

What about people getting their basic needs met? These are called the determinants of wellbeing, and much of this contributes specifically to mental wellbeing too. So things like having an income that affords some kind of liveable quality of life, being able to get good quality food, water, sanitation, warm and dry housing, safety, and employment.

People who were already experiencing hardship or poverty and who now may face additional and compounding hardships due to job loss, reduced household income and a broader economic downturn, may find themselves increasingly vulnerable. For many, loss of work can mean loss of social connection, identity, and sense of belonging, and this will be experienced differently according to people's individual circumstances. And addressing things like the precariousness of modern life, where things like housing and employment can't be counted upon, where they may end or change quickly, without much ability to accumulate resources, like money, to get you through lean times.

Additionally, people who perhaps find themselves jobless or with severely reduced incomes for the first time in their lives may find themselves exposed to new high stress levels. This may be coupled with a lack of knowledge about how to obtain support, or associated with stigma about being forced to do so by life circumstances. Support agencies and institutions may not yet have a good grip on how to best help this new group of people.

Secondary stressors typically last a long time and for some people the impact and duration of secondary stressors may be greater than the event itself. These unresolved issues can cause emotional strain and hinder people from rebuilding lives, livelihoods, routines and community. Secondary stressors can contribute to mental health challenges, like sleep problems, fatigue, experiences of trauma, loss and grief, as well as problems related to alcohol and drug use, and excessive gambling. Relationship problems may increase, including the risk of serious harm from family and sexual violence in our communities (particularly accruing to women and children), as well as issues related to broader social cohesion, such as increased racism and other forms of discrimination and marginalisation.

While these effects can be very serious, it is important to view secondary stressors through the lens of 'Problems of Living'. Many people won't directly experience mental distress. It is much more likely that they will be worried about paying bills, rent, mortgages, other outstanding debt, and having enough food to eat, clothes to wear, and money for transport, power and heating — and that's what worries them, causes anxiety and pushes them to behave in unhelpful ways.

In these cases, it also doesn't make sense to treat the anxiety in isolation. It makes far more sense to address the problems that are causing the anxiety and worry. So addressing housing, safety, food, water, income support, employment and providing support to those who provide employment and income-generating opportunities for others. All this needs to run alongside ramping up services to help those who need support in dealing with the anxiety they feel.

If we focus our support on dealing with 'Problems of Living', then we've a good chance of helping people with their living circumstances as well as dealing with the very real discomfort and worry they may be experiencing right now.

Measuring the impact of secondary stressors

Tracking the impacts of secondary stressors is not easy, as there may be unintended consequences of policy decisions that may not start showing their impact until substantial numbers of people are affected. However, some broad measures can give us a clue as to what is happening.

One of these is a measure of economic activity: GDP. If we look at GDP as a broad measure of the economic impacts of both Covid-19 and the measures taken by various governments to manage its impact and spread, we can see that they are considerable and have a very real impact on people's sense of economic wellbeing.

But is growth, or the distinct shrinking of it as captured by GDP figures, everything? Critics have noted that GDP is not a great measure of 'the economy'. GDP only captures 'market transactions': it ignores the value and contributions of voluntary and unpaid labour. The contributions of many of those 'essential workers' such as supermarket staff are valued at not much more than the minimum wage. GDP rates the value of bond traders much higher than laboratory technicians. Life preservation and also the impacts of what has been called long-Covid also need to be taken into account.

What is not accounted for is the counterfactual: what would be the costs if we did as a few people have suggested and let the virus 'run through' the population? Let alone the death rate, and serious long-term health impacts on those infected, what would it do to psychological wellbeing, confidence in the economy, and people's work productivity?

These are hard to measure, and for some intolerable to think about, but when people criticise the public health measures that have been implemented, I believe that they have not fully thought through the alternatives, or indeed have proposed any meaningful, fully worked-through alternative measures that can be scrutinised, stress-tested and considered. There simply aren't any alternative workable solutions that address the deadly dilemma of fulfilling the fundamental task of government: to protect the life and wellbeing of its citizens.

As we progress through our pandemic journey, it's clear that the secondary impacts of the measures taken to protect the wellbeing of populations around the world will vary according to each government's policies. These secondary stressors will be experienced differently, and have different outcomes. Indeed, the lack of clear policy decisions, or confused messaging can also have secondary impacts and may be stressors in and of themselves.

Whatever the cause, managing the impacts of these secondary stressors will be among the biggest challenge as we emerge from lockdowns and start to regularise international connections through trade and travel. It may also present our greatest opportunity for economic transformation to address other existential threats that we have been reluctant to grasp, namely the threat and impact of climate change. How and when we decide to take this opportunity is in our hands.

CASE STUDY: Living with prolonged stress in the aftermath of the Canterbury earthquakes

From 2010 to 2017, I was involved in providing psychosocial advice and support to government bodies in the wake of the Canterbury earthquakes, in New Zealand. Indeed, this work continues now and again, particularly around significant anniversaries and milestones. This extended earthquake sequence offers many lessons in terms of how it mirrors Covid-19 in its sudden and seemingly unexpected nature, and the extended mental health impacts and economic ramifications of the event.

On 22 February 2011 at 12.51pm, New Zealand's Canterbury region was struck by a magnitude 6.3 earthquake. The region was still recovering from a magnitude 7.1 earthquake, which struck just over five months earlier, on 4 September 2010.

While New Zealand is sometimes known as the 'Shaky Isles' due to its location at the convergence of two major tectonic plates, the initial Canterbury earthquake came completely out of the blue for a region previously considered low risk (though Māori had indigenous knowledge of previous earthquakes in the region). After being shaken awake in the early hours of 4 September, there was a wide sense of relief among residents of the region's capital Christchurch that the city had 'dodged a bullet'.

In fact, the story was just beginning. The 22 February 2011 earthquake caused greater devastation in most parts of the region. Although smaller than the first quake, and technically part of its aftershock sequence, the timing, shallow depth and proximity of the epicentre to the central city meant that the February earthquake was more destructive. The earthquake flattened much of the central business district, several major buildings collapsed and 185 lives were lost.

With further major earthquakes in February, June and December 2011 and a total of more than 10,000 aftershocks, Cantabrians lived with ongoing stress and uncertainty for more than two years and many for much longer. Jobs were lost, businesses folded, and there was an anxious wait to find out which homes, or indeed entire neighbourhoods, would be 'red zoned' and condemned. Families experienced financial stress, difficulties with insurance and rebuilding, and anxiety about sending their kids to school each day or committing to major projects with the ever present and unpredictable threat of another major quake.

Things would seem to be getting back to normal again, when

another quake or aftershock would strike in an unexpected place, seemingly unrelated to the previous earthquake shock. Yet again people would find themselves thrown into uncertainty, with lives and livelihoods threatened, and imagined or actual future life trajectories disrupted.

Can you see the parallels with Covid-19?

In the first year of the pandemic, there have been repeated outbreaks of various scale in different regions of the world, varying from localised outbreaks to rampant contagion practically unchecked over several waves of infection, even taking hold again in countries where the number of infected cases and affected people were trending downwards. The pandemic is likely to carry on deep into its second year before there is any hope of effective vaccines being distributed and taken up by enough of the global population to bring virus spread under any kind of control. And in some areas of the world, it could take considerably longer.

So what can we learn from what happened in Canterbury and over the subsequent decade, that can help to inform us in dealing with other crises and prolonged periods of uncertainty, like that which we are now facing?

While several studies have been carried out regarding mental health impacts of the earthquakes, the majority were completed less than two years after the onset of the earthquake sequence. This means that we know relatively little about delayed or persistent responses and whether initial effects have decreased over the following 10 years. This is why it may be more useful to look at accumulated evidence and trends, rather than focusing on short-term impacts or single studies.

The best overview of the literature suggests that for most crisis events, around 80% of people will adjust successfully so long as they remain socially connected, have adequate financial resources, safe housing, and can get their basic needs met; 10–15% will require ongoing support through counselling or family doctor level services; while 5–10% of those exposed to the crisis may need intensive psychological support.

As for kids in Canterbury, the largest study looked at the emotional and behaviour scores from the universal before-school check and did not detect any evidence of negative impacts from the earthquake. The same goes for elders. The only study focused on older adults did not report significant differences between those exposed to the earthquakes and those who were not.

While a small percentage of adults will need ongoing support, there is a growing body of evidence from Canterbury that some people experience post-traumatic growth following individual and collective adversity. The experience of going through the earthquakes meant that some people recalibrated and readjusted their lives towards more meaningful and purposeful activity that reflected what they wanted out of life, rather than carrying on as before.

In this sense, the break in life's trajectory didn't mean an inexorable downwards path to despair and poor mental health. Rather, it was taken as an opportunity — albeit negotiated and adjusted over a period of time — to a new trajectory that reflected their new circumstances of life, leading to a different and improved level of satisfaction and wellbeing.

Another study from Canterbury showed that a sense of control, agency and self-determination can enhance people's wellbeing.[2]

2. Thornley, L, Ball, J, Signal, L, Lawson-Te Aho, K, & Rawson, E (2013). Building

That's why it's so important that we involve people and community organisations in the response to a crisis. When people sense that they have a stake in the outcome, and that these shared outcomes are created collaboratively and collectively, then they are much more likely to 'buy in' and contribute towards making that outcome a reality. This creates the possibility of a virtuous circle, where individual wellbeing is enhanced by community resilience and vice versa.

Many people commented that the fact that their communities felt very well connected before the earthquakes helped them to adapt afterwards. Pre-existing networks — including online channels — were important. In all communities studied, participants reported a post-earthquake increase in community connectedness, especially in the immediate aftermath and 'honeymoon period', when people acted selflessly and were more caring and generous than usual.

There were also negative impacts such as damage to housing and loss of public facilities, which led to the displacement of residents and disruption to the fabric of community cohesion. Some found themselves tending to stay at home due to fear of impending aftershocks, which is perhaps reminiscent of behaviour during the Covid-19 pandemic where there has been a reluctance by some to emerge into community activity because they have been advised to self-isolate, or they have determined themselves that the risk of contagion is larger than they are prepared to bear.

In the immediate aftermath of the Christchurch earthquakes, many people were unable to contribute to community action. From aftershocks to housing issues, difficulty accessing support, and general uncertainty, many experienced chronic stress, depression,

Community Resilience: Learning from the Canterbury Earthquakes. Research Report. March 2013. New Zealand.

anxiety and fatigue. Once people were able to contribute, they often reported regaining energy and improved wellbeing. This meant they had more energy to contribute to these community initiatives, and so the virtuous circle continued.

That's why taking care of our communities is so important, both before and after a crisis. Where opportunities to connect are restricted, and community facilities are closed or otherwise out of action, that reduces the capacity of the community to cope with the challenges. In this Covid-19 world we must plan to bolster community connection, or face a bumpier path to recovery.

CHAPTER 12

The lockdown yo-yo

If you're lucky, by now you've had a period of time where restrictions have eased. Hopefully you have been able to get on with life, more or less as normal. You didn't have to think about every little action and you didn't have to worry so much, so you may have been able to let go of some of that anxiety. Maybe you've even become a little complacent with things like hand washing and physical distancing.

Philosophers call this feeling of stability our sense of ontological security[1] and it hinges on three factors:

1. A stable sense of home,
2. A feeling that nature is benign, or, at least, not out to get us, and
3. A sense that our contract with society and our fellow citizens is not harmful and preferably positive.

When you've experienced a time of relative freedom, hearing that the virus has escalated and we have to move back into restrictions or lockdown again can come as a real shock. It knocks our confidence in the systems that are supposed to ensure our safety, like border controls and contact tracing, especially if mistakes have been made. It turns out that we are less safe than we had thought,

---

1. Giddens, A (1991). *Modernity and Self-Identity: Self and Society in the Late Modern Age*. California: Stanford University Press.

and so our threat system experiences this as real and present danger, even if the actual risk remains small.

That can bring up all sorts of emotions. You might feel shock and bewilderment, or a sense of dread. *Here we go again.* You might feel frozen or paralysed by the threat of the virus.

Have you ever driven past a car accident? For a moment, the risk of driving is brought to life — not in an abstract way, but in a vivid, tangible and terrible way. You might slow down and take a long look at what happened. You might then drive on, but much more slowly than you were driving before.

But how long does that new behaviour last? I've asked many people this in workshops, and the general answer is a few minutes. For a brief time the accident pierces our protective bubble and threatens our sense of ontological security. But very quickly, our perceptions of invulnerability return and we soon speed up again.

In this way, we are engaged in a constant balancing act — to recognise a risk, but to avoid obsessing about it. To take stock of the possibilities, without allowing awareness of possibilities to stop us from doing what we are doing. We have to build up our capacity to get on with things, or life will completely paralyse us as we check each small detail for risk.

If and when fresh restrictions are announced and you feel that rising dread that indicates your ontological security is threatened, the first step is to take control of your calming system and disengage your threat detection system. This will give you some breathing room so you can make good decisions and judgements. Even though your brain is telling you there is a real and imminent danger, the health risk is still very small, especially if you keep taking basic precautions like following hygiene protocols.

Understandably, with fresh restrictions people will also have a part of their mind focused on the future threat of trying to earn a living, or trying to save their businesses from going under. Governments need to understand that this can become a critical driver of behaviour, so this fear needs to be factored into messaging to help keep people safe as they try to navigate their everyday activities, and also in terms of the practical assistance they may need.

As we have seen in previous crises, it is often these secondary stressors that end up having the bigger impact — and we cannot know what this will look like at the beginning. This does not justify non-intervention into the primary event itself, in this case Covid-19 and the attempts to stop the spread. We will never know what would have happened if we did not make serious attempts to control the spread of the disease, but we can hypothesise that as the health impact would have been exponentially more catastrophic, so would have been the secondary impacts and stress generated by the health impact.

It helps if the authorities can assure us of our safety by fixing any glitches with systems that are out of our control, like border control and quarantine procedures. Once we have confidence that these systems are working well, our minds can stop treating that as a potential threat to our safety and we are more likely to be able to return to our usual activities. We can get caught up in our daily lives again until the next time our attention is drawn to something that triggers our threat detection system.

It's not good when it happens, but mistakes do occur. And unfortunately, these can have consequences that mean the world suddenly feels a lot more unpredictable and uncertain again. It's important that we can be assured that mistakes are being addressed, and that we can get good information about the size and the nature of the actual risk. If these are not addressed, our threat-detecting brains keep racing to protect us against events as if they are life-threatening and this can provoke big emotional reactions.

Embarking on Lockdown 2.0, 3.0, ...

When the virus resurges and lockdown strikes again, how do we go back to staying home to break the chain and save lives? Until we have better treatments and a safe and widely accessible vaccine, we will need to go through a phase of actively reminding ourselves of what we need to do when we act like we have the virus.

The risk of imposing restrictions in subsequent waves is that we can develop a sense of resignation, and that may take two forms: apathy and determination.

Part of this will depend on our earlier experiences of attempts to control the spread and impact of Covid-19. Having a sense of agency — the belief that we, or others who operate on our behalf in the institutions of government, can exert some control and influence over the spread of the virus — may mean that this feeling of resignation is partnered with a sense of determination. We may not like the situation we find ourselves in, but we will act in order to meet the challenge.

However, if our previous experiences were paired with a sense of helplessness and being cast aside and alone to deal with the threat ourselves, and that we were being governed and protected ineffectively, then this is more likely to be paired with a sense of apathy: no matter what we do, it will make no difference to the control of spread and impact of the coronavirus. These are dangerous times, and to a certain extent, locked in through previous experiences.

Concerted action, consistently taken over a period of time by all, can start to change any apathetic view — but it will take time, and a large degree of support, and notable successes to make meaningful changes to this attitude once it starts to take root.

In New Zealand, and in many places around the world where good progress was made in limiting the speed and impact of the coronavirus, we learned that we can experience success, if not elimination. I think we learned that if we could make sure our basic needs were being met – that we had a reliable income and that we could get food — then we could actually get through this.

Along the way, one of the by-products was perhaps a realisation that people weren't overly in love with the lives they were living pre-coronavirus anyway. As they went through lockdown, and if they were in a position to get their basic needs met, they then tried to make changes to take forwards with them into whatever life looked like after lockdown. Perhaps organisations learned that people working at home can still get stuff done. And perhaps people also learned that teaching your kids isn't easy, and trying to do that and work at the same time is, at times, impossible. Teachers, you are the new heroes. Please take all the teacher-only training days you need.

One of the difficulties of lockdown is staying focused on the collective goal and avoiding stay-at-home fatigue. This occurs after a period of restriction, when we start to get cabin fever and feel tempted to break the rules, even if the virus hasn't changed and the risk remains the same. During the initial lockdowns, one study following cellphone data showed that people started going out more frequently and travelling longer distances from home, after they passed that one-month mark of being confined to their home.

It has also been reported that the UK government discussed moving to a seven-day self-isolation period for those exhibiting Covid-19 symptoms — rather than the WHO recommendation of

14 days — because the evidence suggested people were more likely to stick to a seven-day isolation period (versus very low adherence to the 14-day policy). Governments have to deal with stay-at-home fatigue in a range of ways and these shifting sands make it even more difficult for people to understand what they need to do.

One simple explanation for stay-at-home fatigue that has been used by economists is called 'diminishing marginal utility'. During the first few days in lockdown, you probably had the opportunity to do things in the house that you were fairly enthusiastic about. Maybe you binge-watched Netflix, or built a blanket fort with your kids. But after several weeks at home your kids are driving you nuts, you're tired of trying to direct their learning, you're into the dregs of Netflix shows and you just want it to stop.

In other words, you've used up all the 'high utility' (i.e. high happiness) activities and are now scraping the bottom of the barrel. Cue stay-at-home fatigue, and the creeping desire to get out.

Many of us also appear to be driven by what it called 'idleness aversion'. This may be a conditioned thing that we've grown to expect in life, but briefly, it's our desire to get out of the house and do something, whether it's a visit with friends or a trip to the burger place that's more a craving than a necessity. Research shows that we don't actually like sitting around and doing nothing for extended periods of time all that much. One study found that when subjects were told to sit in a room and do nothing, they chose to give themselves electric shocks rather than pass the time in silence.

So how can we motivate ourselves to stick to the rules? In conditions of uncertainty, or when we are not entirely sure how to act or what to think, we look to others for cues on what we should be doing. This is where we all need to act as leaders. To practise physical distancing, to wear a mask if we can. To wash our hands. To remain kind and courteous to others, even though this might be a big inconvenience in our lives. Remember that the goal is the return to some kind of normal living, bar the international travel, as soon as possible and this is only going to happen if we all play our part.

Unfortunately, looking to others can also play out in the opposite direction to our goals. The more we witness people breaking the rules and regulations with little perceived cost, the more likely it is that we will also be tempted to breach rules and regulations: *If everyone else is doing it, why can't I do it too?*

Be realistic and intentional about what you need to do to play your part. Work hard on your wellbeing. We can still be civil, adopt the appropriate manners for our situation, and wait it out. It's hard to remain physically distant, but it's something we may need to maintain for a while longer.

We've done this before, so we know we can do it again. We're also depending on each other to do the right thing and it's only going to work if we do this together. But small actions by determined individuals can quickly add up to create a movement, and to signal to others through our actions that what we do matters and can make a difference.

Here's how to strengthen your resolve and get through:

1. Reduce the overwhelm. You've done this before, you can do this again. Think about what worked for you last time and do more of that.

2. Make a public promise. If this fits with you, tell people what you are doing. When you go public with your intentions, it immediately strengthens your resolve, so announce it to friends and family on Facebook or by email. A public commitment shifts your own thinking about your seriousness. No one wants to be embarrassed in front of others.

3. Set up accountability partners. Recruit people like you to help you stay the course and build each other's resolve. Create a system of accountability so that you can report your actions, successes and failures every day. This may be a friend or it could be on Facebook, or in a forum of some kind. Don't just announce it once and then disappear; let the world know about your progress, and your successes.

4. Expect difficulties. There will be life situations that might get in the way of your efforts and it is so easy to allow them to undermine all your hard work. Think in advance of possible problems that might arise and decide how you will deal with these situations and how you can stick to the plan.

5. Think of the consequences. Another way to strengthen your resolve is to think of the consequences before you take an action that will lead to them. Not just for you, but for everyone and all the effort that's been put in so far. Pondering consequences certainly isn't a magic pill, but it can help if you usually don't think about the consequences until they become real. Because that will most likely be too late.

6. Imagine others you respect can see you. Last but most definitely not least, you can benefit from some social pressure. Next time you want to choose the easy way out, imagine other people whose opinion you respect can see you. Would you still take that unnecessary trip if they could see you? And what would disapproval from them feel like to you? Yes, you're essentially manipulating yourself, but if it works to strengthen your resolve to stick with a course of action that you value right now, then it's certainly a tool you can go to.

Persistent anxiety

Just as our experiences of lockdown are different, so are our experiences of re-emerging into society again. Some may experience a sense of persistent anxiety as they return to a more social life. This may take the form of not wanting to get too close to other people, a lingering sense of dread, being easily distracted, poor sleep, or other physiological signs.

Some may even experience a wider sense of risk aversion in the short term. We may find ourselves avoiding places, activities or situations, or worrying excessively about issues outside our control.

Underlying all this is a need for certainty that isn't being met, and is unlikely to be met for some time, together with a belief that more information will help to relieve anxiety and worry. Unfortunately, many outcomes in life are unpredictable, or can't be predicted with absolute certainty. Assuming that certainty is possible actually keeps anxiety going.

So why might anxiety persist post-lockdown? Being asked to pivot from a mindset of acting like we have coronavirus and avoiding all unnecessary contact, to being able to be near people again (albeit with physical distancing measures) is a big shift. We are moving from a situation where there was a widely shared model of what was happening and how we should respond, to a new phase, where there may be different ideas about what is and is not appropriate.

Children and younger adults may need guidance as to how to behave, but also dealing with the emotions it may raise for them; feeling a sense of psychological danger. We know that for the best learning to take place we need structure and predictability, but we also need to feel psychologically safe, so that our cognitive space isn't taken up with thoughts of worry, and that we aren't too caught up in the emotional labour and hard work of managing these silent emotions ourselves.

Moving back into society can also bring us face to face with the social and economic consequences in ways that we may not have been in touch with in real ways thus far: job losses, business closures or furloughs. This may bring up feelings of shame, loss and guilt.

As restrictions ease, we can also be faced with a deluge of information. Instead of tuning in to government press conferences, we are bombarded with info from clubs, schools, shops, cafés, councils. We may even end up with conflicting information, which creates doubt and more uncertainty. Some things might get overlooked completely — and when we search for some piece of information we need and find that no one has said anything about it, again, this can erode our sense of psychological safety.

Now some people like more information — it settles them. Others want to be told what they need to do directly and from one source only. And, of course, there is every possible variation in between.

It's important to remember that for most people, this low-grade and possibly persistent anxiety will most likely not interfere with their lives, and it will most likely fade away and flare up only when we go through another concerning period if cases start rising again. It's only when anxiety is so strong that it interferes with your being able to carry out your normal day-to-day life, that it is considered to be an anxiety disorder.

It's also likely we will start to normalise some of the behaviours that we have been encouraged to perform, like washing hands more often and physical distancing. These will become a way of life for the foreseeable future, and will have consequences for interactions and relationships that are hard to project right now.

We need to keep observing, experiencing, and understanding that we have a diversity of emerging needs that won't be fully apparent just yet. When we first start emerging into social spaces, like school or the workplace, there might be a level of comfort you need to feel safe. It's important that schools and workplaces respect this and help people to manage safe interactions — not just infection safe, but *psychologically* safe. This means that people will be able to go at their own pace, and it will likely add another dimension to getting back to social life.

In terms of schools, I have some sympathy for the view that children need the structure of getting back to school. But creating a sense of psychological safety is also paramount if the learning opportunities that the schooling system provides are going to be effectively taken up.

Parents also need to understand what they need to do at the school gate etc. in order to keep them safe. While we can't eliminate the possibility of the virus spreading among children when they are mixing freely, it's how we prepare and react to this that becomes important. And it is important that if you are sick, you stay at home.

The good news is that there is a way out of this cycle of looking for certainty. Instead of trying to control things or block out your thoughts and feelings, you can learn how to experience them in a manageable way.

Anxiety is a normal human emotion when faced with threat, but some people will find that everyday things start to feel like a threat and anxiety begins to limit your day-to-day life. In this situation, we tend to overestimate how likely it is that something bad will happen to us and underestimate our ability to cope. Here are some tips to help you get some awareness of how your worries and anxiety might be driving your behaviour, so you can start to take action to feel more in charge, even if you can't get absolute certainty in your life right now.

- **Get to know your anxiety.** Keep a diary of when it's at its best — and worst. Find the patterns and plan your week, or day, to proactively manage your anxiety.
- **Know that everyone experiences anxiety.** It is a normal human response to situations that may include some kind of threat, real or perceived. It can help you to prepare well for big events and to take care in situations that objectively are risky. It's important to expect and learn to tolerate some anxiety, but it's also important to recognise when your anxiety has become unhelpful and take action to counter it.
- **Learn from others.** Talking with others who also experience anxiety — or are going through something similar — can help you feel less alone.
- **Try graded exposure.** Taking small steps to face the thing you are worried about and build your confidence to cope is called graded exposure. When you face a fear by doing the thing you've been avoiding, your fight or flight response will be triggered. But if you stay long enough in the situation you are worried about, your fight or flight response — and therefore your anxiety — goes down. Usually you will find that your fear was unfounded, which is an empowering experience. If you keep doing it a bit more or staying a bit longer each time, your anxiety still rises at the start each time, but not as much as the time before. When you do the thing that worries you again and again, your anxiety goes away faster each time. Eventually, you find that you can do much more than before, without being worried about it.
- **Finally, be kind to yourself.** Remember that you are not your anxiety. You are not weak. You are not inferior. Take small acts of bravery. Avoiding what makes you anxious provides some

relief in the short term, but can make you more anxious in the long term. Try approaching something that makes you anxious — even in a small way. The way through anxiety is by learning that what you fear isn't likely to happen — and if it does, you'll be able to cope with it.

Anxiety about going out

Whereas during lockdown some people may have experienced FOMO, or fear of missing out, anxiety about life after lockdown shows up for some people as FOGO, or fear of going out.

Even though 'lockdown' may be incredibly hard for people to comply with, there's no doubt that for many, it offers that increased sense of safety. At its core, FOGO is about the balance people are experiencing between that sense of safety and the uncertainty they feel about the world outside of their safe spaces, and how that safety will be managed 'out there'.

During lockdown periods we are deluged with information from governments and the media telling us to stay inside as much as possible to control the spread of coronavirus. We have to figure out whether it was safe to go for a walk or a run, to go to the shop to get food, how to make sure we stayed far enough apart from other people. We have to adapt to a new way of life — not just for a few days, but for weeks at a time.

This is where FOGO may have been born. In a very real sense, it's very closely tied to a threat. We feel at risk of perhaps being infected by the virus, and we feel vulnerable. So we take steps to protect ourselves. And one way in which that has become embedded in our behaviour is through staying at home.

You don't have to live in a place with lots of coronavirus cases to feel anxious about going out after a period of restriction. And the problem is that unless we are careful and strategic about changing our behaviour, then it becomes not just embedded (meaning a behaviour that we are used to, and we can choose to behave in that way, or not) but entrenched. When a behaviour is entrenched it becomes our automatic response, so that when we don't behave in a way that we feel keeps us safe (staying inside), the feelings of vulnerability and accompanying anxiety threaten to overwhelm us.

As we move forward and learn to live with the virus, we have to balance the risks between becoming overly concerned about catching Covid-19 and the effects that the pandemic will have on wider society in the next few months and years. People's livelihoods depend upon economic activity. Even if we are buying things online, it doesn't replace full economic activity and the flow-on effects for business viability and job security.

Of course, there are other things going on in the world right now which could mean that you're wise to stay at home to keep yourself safe — there's no denying that. But as far as the pandemic goes, if you don't have a pre-existing condition that puts you at risk of severe impacts of Covid-19, or you're not in the potentially vulnerable older adults group, then the risk of the economy falling over then starts to become something you probably need to pay attention to because, ultimately, this affects you too.

That's why we need to recalibrate our assessment of risk to include not just the health risk, but the risks of other societal impacts — including your safety behaviour becoming so entrenched that it becomes even harder to change in the longer term. Multiply that by thousands of people being fearful of going out and you can see how this can have a big impact on society as a whole.

The key to managing all this is to remain flexible. To be able to stay home when disease spread is a real risk, but then to be able to emerge and re-engage with society when those disease risks become manageable for most people. Rather than thinking of your current circumstances as a 'new normal', with the predictability that this implies, it's probably better to prepare ourselves for more change, as businesses and organisations grapple with the prospect of ongoing changes over a number of months and years.

So how can you bring yourself to go out when people say that it's safe, but it doesn't *feel* safe to you? Our understanding of a specific type of phobia called agoraphobia can be helpful here. Agoraphobia is a fear of going out and it is a reaction to an actual or anticipated situation that is perceived as difficult or impossible to escape. This also then gives us a clue as to what we might be able to do about FOGO.

If your agoraphobia isn't too overwhelming, then it's important that you face your fear by going out often, so that the fear doesn't grow. The more often we let a fear stop us from doing something, the harder it is to do it the next time. The key is to feel the fear and don't let it stop you doing things. As the saying goes: Feel that fear, and do it anyway.

If your agoraphobia is stronger, you can ask family and friends to come with you when you go out. Let them know in advance that you might have to wait for a panic attack to pass, or even go home so that you feel less pressured or embarrassed if that happens. That's okay. It might take a few goes before this starts working for you. But don't get discouraged. Try to stay out for a bit longer each time you try to go out.

Exercise can help. If you can, go outside for a walk each day, especially in a nature environment like the park, the beach or a bush, forest or river trail. If you are housebound, it's still important to move as much as possible. Even just getting used to being outdoors again is a step in the right direction.

More generally, we humans can find change difficult. Being asked to change direction again after being asked to stay inside might take some getting used to, so places might feel more empty than usual for a while after restrictions ease. On the other hand, those people who adapt quickly are likely to throng to the places that are actually open for business, perhaps making them feel more crowded than usual. That can be off-putting if it's your first foray back into re-engaging with society, so be aware of those possible false impressions too and try to take that into account. As restrictions start to open up more widely, people usually start to spread out a bit more naturally again in open society — but expect that to take a bit of time.

You don't suddenly have to throw yourself out into the deep end. It is a gradual process and you can do it at your own pace. We humans are social beings, but we also have our own needs for safety and to feel like we have individual control too. If it feels like a step too far, then take your time.

Dealing with quarantine

One important tool for limiting the spread and impact of Covid-19 is the implementation of various forms of managed isolation and quarantine (MIQ) arrangements around the world. When people cross borders between nations, or even between states in the case of Australia, they have been required to spend up to 14 days in managed isolation facilities, sometimes at their own expense. For many people, this is a difficult experience.

Quarantine is the separation and restriction of movement of people who have potentially been exposed to a contagious disease to see if they become unwell, so reducing the risk of them infecting others. Isolation is the separation of people who have been diagnosed with a contagious disease from people who are not sick. The two terms are often used interchangeably and this could be a possible point of confusion for those entering 'managed isolation' facilities, and for the public.

While we know something about the psychological impact for people with symptoms who are separated from others to reduce infection risk (isolation), we know relatively little about the psychological impacts for those who may have been exposed to the virus resulting in possible infection, but their viral/disease status has not yet been confirmed (quarantine).

Research from previous disease outbreaks shows that when people go into quarantine, factors such as separation from loved ones, loss of freedom, uncertainty over disease status and boredom can have big impacts. Suicide has been reported in the research, people experience substantial anger, and legal action has been taken following the imposition of quarantine following outbreaks of other diseases, such as SARS. The evidence seems to point to the imposition of a restriction of liberty being at the root of this; because voluntary quarantine is associated with less distress and fewer long-term complications.

In the case of Covid-19 in New Zealand, quarantine stress may have been made worse by difficult circumstances leading up to arrival in the country, including financial distress, multiple cancellations of flights with long waits for further availability, immigration and visa issues in the country from which they were returning, and negative media coverage, including social media — producing a feeling that returnees are unwelcome in their own country, even if they are returning for reasons such as the impending death of a loved one.

If we look at the experiences of people quarantined during previous

SARS outbreaks,[2] over 20% reported fear, 18% reported nervousness, 18% reported sadness, and 10% reported guilt. They also had experiences like grief,[3] numbness,[4] and anxiety-induced insomnia.[5]

During the equine influenza outbreak in Australia,[6] people were quarantined for several weeks because of that disease outbreak — and 34% of horse owners who were quarantined reported high levels of psychological distress, compared with around 12% in the general Australian population.

We know that quarantine is stressful, and it is linked to people experiencing a number of different and difficult worries and emotions, with sometimes serious consequences. So why is quarantine so hard? The difficulties experienced appear to fall into five categories:

1. Duration of quarantine

Some studies have shown that longer durations of quarantine were associated with poorer mental health, post-traumatic stress

2. Reynolds, DL, Garay, JR, Deamond, SL, Moran, MK, Gold, W, & Styra, R (2008). Understanding, compliance and psychological impact of the SARS quarantine experience. *Epidemiol Infect*, 136:997–1007.
3. Wang, Y, Xu, B, Zhao, G, Cao, R, He, X, & Fu, S. (2011). Is quarantine related to immediate negative psychological consequences during the 2009 H1N1 epidemic? *Gen Hosp Psychiatry*, 33:75–77.
4. Pan, PJD, Chang, S-H, & Yu, Y-Y. (2005). A support group for home-quarantined college students exposed to SARS: learning from practice. *J Spec Group Work*, 30:363–374.
5. DiGiovanni, C, Conley, J, Chiu, D, & Zaborski, J. (2004). Factors influencing compliance with quarantine in Toronto during the 2003 SARS outbreak. *Biosecur Bioterror*, 2:265–272.
6. Taylor, MR, Agho, KE, Stevens, GJ, & Raphael, B. (2008). Factors influencing psychological distress during a disease epidemic: data from Australia's first outbreak of equine influenza. *BMC Public Health*, 8:347.

symptoms,[7] avoidance behaviours, and anger.[8] Although the duration of the quarantine was not always clear, one study showed that those quarantined for more than 10 days showed significantly higher post-traumatic stress symptoms than those quarantined for fewer than 10 days.[9]

2. Fears of infection

Participants in many studies reported fears about their own health and were more likely to fear infecting family members or others, than those not quarantined. They also became particularly worried if they experienced any physical symptoms potentially related to the infection, and these worries and other psychological symptoms could continue for months.[10]

3. Frustration and boredom

Confinement, loss of usual routine, and reduced social and physical contact with others were frequently shown to cause boredom, frustration, and a sense of isolation from the rest of the world, which was distressing to participants.[11] This frustration was made

7. Hawryluck, L, Gold, WL, Robinson, S, Pogorski, S, Galea, S, & Styra, R. (2004). SARS control and psychological effects of quarantine, Toronto, Canada. *Emerg Infect Dis*, 10:1206–1212.

8. Marjanovic, Z, Greenglass, ER, & Coffey, S. (2007). The relevance of psychosocial variables and working conditions in predicting nurses' coping strategies during the SARS crisis: an online questionnaire survey. *Int J Nurs Stud*, 44:991–998.

9. Hawryluck, L, Gold, WL, Robinson, S, Pogorski, S, Galea, S, & Styra, R. (2004). SARS control and psychological effects of quarantine, Toronto, Canada. *Emerg Infect Dis*, 10:1206–1212.

10. Jeong, H, Yim, HW, Song, Y-J, et al. (2016). Mental health status of people isolated due to Middle East respiratory syndrome. *Epidemiol Health*, 38: e2016048.

11. Many studies but e.g. again: Hawryluck, L, Gold, WL, Robinson, S, Pogorski, S, Galea, S, & Styra, R. (2004). SARS control and psychological effects of quarantine, Toronto, Canada. *Emerg Infect Dis*, 10: 1206–1212.

worse by not being able to take part in usual day-to-day activities, such as shopping for basic necessities,[12] or taking part in social networking activities via the telephone or internet.[13] The ability to get outdoors to exercise and exposure to natural light and surroundings also possibly falls into this category too.

4. Inadequate supplies

Having inadequate basic supplies (e.g. food, water, clothes, or accommodation) during quarantine was a source of frustration[14] and continued to be associated with anxiety and anger four to six months after release.[15] Being unable to get regular medical care and prescriptions also appeared to be a problem for some participants. Four studies found that supplies from public health authorities were insufficient. Participants reported receiving their masks and thermometers late or not at all;[16] food, water, and other items were only intermittently distributed; and food supplies took a long time to arrive.[17]

12. Hawryluck, L, Gold, WL, Robinson, S, Pogorski, S, Galea, S, & Styra, R. (2004). SARS control and psychological effects of quarantine, Toronto, Canada. *Emerg Infect Dis*, 10:1206–1212.

13. Jeong, H, Yim, HW, Song, Y-J, et al. (2016). Mental health status of people isolated due to Middle East respiratory syndrome. *Epidemiol Health*, 38: e2016048.

14. Blendon, RJ, Benson, JM, DesRoches, CM, Raleigh, E, & Taylor-Clark, K. (2004). The public's response to severe acute respiratory syndrome in Toronto and the United States. *Clin Infect Dis*, 38:925–931.

15. Jeong, H, Yim, HW, Song, Y-J, et al. (2016). Mental health status of people isolated due to Middle East respiratory syndrome. *Epidemiol Health*, 38: e2016048.

16. Cava, MA, Fay, KE, Beanlands, HJ, McCay, EA, & Wignall, R. (2005). The experience of quarantine for individuals affected by SARS in Toronto. *Public Health Nurs*, 22:398–406.

17. Caleo, G, Duncombe, J, Jephcott, F, et al. (2018). The factors affecting household transmission dynamics and community compliance with Ebola control measures: a mixed-methods study in a rural village in Sierra Leone. *BMC Public Health*, 18:248.

5. Inadequate information

Many participants cited poor information from public health authorities as a stressor, reporting insufficient clear guidelines about actions to take and confusion about the purpose of quarantine.[18] After the Toronto SARS epidemic, participants perceived that confusion stemmed from the differences in style, approach and content of various public health messages because of poor coordination between the multiple jurisdictions and levels of government involved.[19] Lack of clarity about the different levels of risk in particular, led to participants fearing the worst.[20]

What about when people leave quarantine? What's likely to make things worse after they complete their required time?

1. Finances

Financial loss can be a problem during quarantine, with people unable to work or having to interrupt their professional activities with no advance planning — and perhaps having been in limbo for weeks or months before entering quarantine when they cross an international border. The effects appear to be long lasting. The evidence is that financial loss as a result of quarantine created serious socio-economic distress and was found to be a risk factor

18. Many studies, but e.g. again: Cava, MA, Fay, KE, Beanlands, HJ, McCay, EA, & Wignall, R. (2005). The experience of quarantine for individuals affected by SARS in Toronto. *Public Health Nurs*, 22:398–406.
19. DiGiovanni, C, Conley, J, Chiu, D, & Zaborski, J. (2004). Factors influencing compliance with quarantine in Toronto during the 2003 SARS outbreak. *Biosecur Bioterror*, 2:265–272.
20. Desclaux, A, Badji, D, Ndione, AG, & Sow, K. (2017). Accepted monitoring or endured quarantine? Ebola contacts' perceptions in Senegal. *Soc Sci Med*, 178:38–45.

for symptoms of psychological disorders[21] and both anger and anxiety several months after quarantine.[22]

2. Stigma

Stigma from others, often continuing for some time after quarantine, even after containment of the outbreak, is a major issue. In a comparison of healthcare workers quarantined versus those not quarantined, quarantined participants were significantly more likely to report stigmatisation and rejection from people in their local neighbourhoods,[23] suggesting that there is stigma specifically surrounding people who had been quarantined.

General education about the disease and the reasons for quarantine and public health information provided to the general public can help to reduce stigmatisation — and that includes through the media too. Because it is certainly possible that media reporting contributes to stigmatising attitudes in the general public; the media is a powerful influence on public attitudes, and dramatic headlines and fear-mongering have been shown to contribute to stigmatising attitudes in the past (e.g. during the SARS outbreak[24]).

So what can we do to protect people from the most psychologically

21. Mihashi, M, Otsubo, Y, Yinjuan, X, Nagatomi, K, Hoshiko, M, & Ishitake, T. (2009). Predictive factors of psychological disorder development during recovery following SARS outbreak. *Health Psychol*, 28:91–100.
22. Jeong, H, Yim, HW, Song, Y-J, et al. (2016). Mental health status of people isolated due to Middle East respiratory syndrome. *Epidemiol Health*, 38: e2016048.
23. Bai, Y, Lin, C-C, Lin, C-Y, Chen, J-Y, Chue, C-M, & Chou, P. (2004). Survey of stress reactions among health care workers involved with the SARS outbreak. *Psychiatr Serv*, 55:1055–1057.
24. Person, B, Sy, F, Holton, K, et al. (2004). Fear and stigma: the epidemic within the SARS outbreak. *Emerg Infect Dis*, 10:358–363.

damaging aspects of being in quarantine, and what happens afterwards?

1. Keep it as short as possible

Longer quarantine is associated with worse psychological outcomes; the longer the stressor was experienced, the bigger effect it seemed to have. Evidence from elsewhere also emphasises the importance of authorities adhering to their own recommended length of quarantine, and not extending it. For people already in quarantine, an extension, no matter how small, is likely to make any sense of frustration or demoralisation worse.

2. Give people as much information as possible

People who are quarantined often fear being infected or infecting others. They also often have catastrophic ideas about any physical symptoms experienced during the quarantine period. This fear is a common occurrence for people exposed to a worrying infectious disease, and might be made worse by the often inadequate information people have reported receiving from public health officials leaving them unclear about the risks they faced and why they were being quarantined at all. Ensuring that those under quarantine have a good understanding of the disease in question, and the reasons for quarantine, should be a priority.

3. Reduce the boredom and improve the communication

Boredom and isolation will cause distress; people who are quarantined should be advised about what they can do to ward off boredom and provided with practical advice on coping and stress management techniques. It is also important that public health officials maintain clear lines of communication with people quarantined about what to do if they experience any symptoms, including mental health concerns. A phone line or online service specifically set up for those in quarantine, and staffed by healthcare workers who can provide instructions about what to do in the event of developing illness symptoms, would help reassure people that they will be cared for if they become ill. This service would show those who are quarantined that they have not been forgotten and that their health needs are just as important as those of the wider public.

Reassurance like this could decrease feelings such as fear, worry, and anger. An active outreach strategy, that is health services reaching out to those quarantined proactively rather than reactively waiting to be contacted, can ensure safety and create a sense of being cared for. We should not leave it to the people who are being quarantined to make the first move. Daily check-ins should be the thing.

The psychological impacts of quarantine are wide-ranging and can be long lasting too. I'm not suggesting that quarantine shouldn't be used; the psychological effects of not using quarantine and allowing disease to spread would be worse. However, depriving people of their liberty for the wider public good is contentious and needs to be handled very carefully. If quarantine is essential, then the research suggests that officials should take every measure to ensure that this experience is as tolerable as possible for people.

This can be achieved by: telling people what is happening and why, explaining how long it will continue, providing meaningful activities for them to do while in quarantine, providing clear communication, ensuring basic supplies (such as food, water, and medical supplies) are available, and reinforcing the sense of altruism that people should be experiencing.

And that goes for letting the general public know about this sacrifice too — yes, the public may have already gone through deprivations and sacrifice too — so that message needs to be carefully calibrated, but it's a necessary step to help to ensure that people feel included and not so stigmatised once they emerge from quarantine. Knowing what we now know about quarantine, perhaps we can greet returning citizens with compassion for their experience.

CHAPTER 13

Living with Covid-19

If you think back to the first time that you were asked to change your behaviour drastically and go into 'lockdown', perhaps you remember feeling fear and anxiety. Perhaps you also felt a sense of excitement, a feeling of adventure about this big unknown. There was a newness to it, a 'Blitz spirit', meaning a feeling of coming together to protect each other and try to get on top of the virus. There was hope that this would be a short-term pain until a vaccine emerged, or we found a way to counter the worst effects and lower the risks of severe health outcomes or death. Or we hoped, perhaps silently, that somehow the virus would just ... disappear.

The impact of those initial lockdowns will depend on how you've been affected by those restrictions, and how well you have managed to adapt. For some, control over the knock-on effects of these public health measures was taken completely out of their hands. This is likely to have been the case if you worked in the international tourism industry, or the many businesses that indirectly serve that market. Food suppliers, retailers and other service industries have also been dramatically affected.

For many of the self-employed, or those who employ others, lockdown is a worrying time. Others asked to work in essential services, such as health staff, cleaners, transport and supermarket workers to name but a few, had to balance trying to earn an income while managing personal risks of exposure to the coronavirus and maintaining practices to reduce the risk of unwittingly transmitting the virus to others at home or in other community.

For others, just managing daily tasks with children, other family and household members, getting food and healthcare can be challenging. And still others may have come to value some respite from their usual, perhaps unhealthy, ways of living during the 'lockdown' period.

In some places like New Zealand, Australia, Taiwan, Vietnam and South Korea, we have experienced success. We learned that by acting together, we could drastically reduce or even eliminate the presence of the coronavirus. In other places, it may have felt like an ongoing escalation, a situation spiralling out of control.

As I type this in the middle of November 2020 here in Wellington, New Zealand, I see escalation in numbers and Covid-19 measures all over the world. The World Health Organization's coronavirus dashboard showed a third consecutive daily record high in the number of confirmed new cases. Almost half of those cases were registered in the WHO's Europe region. Italy announced a raft of new restrictions and warned that the country's escalating coronavirus infection rate was already having a worrying impact on hospitals. German authorities reported a record one-day total of new coronavirus cases this weekend and Spain has declared a new nationwide state of emergency in the hope of stemming a resurgence in coronavirus infections. France registered 52,010 new confirmed coronavirus cases in the past week, with daily new case numbers still trending upwards.

In the UK coronavirus has hit hard, with the country recording hundreds of thousands of cases and over 40,000 deaths linked to the disease. England faced Europe's highest excess death levels during the first wave of the pandemic. Case numbers passed the earlier April peak in September and have continued to rise in October, though some of this rise might be attributed to increased levels of testing. England has now embarked upon a further national lockdown for at least 27 days.

US case numbers are still rising to the point where over 12 million Americans have contracted the virus since the pandemic began, and over 250,000 have died. Recent days have seen record-breaking rises in case numbers (and the politically-charged election of a new President).

In Asia, though there are some relative success stories compared with the rest of the world where we have good data, the situation also does not make for good reading. India is closing in on 8 million cases, with 119,000 deaths. China reported detecting 137 new asymptomatic coronavirus cases in Kashgar in the north-western region of Xinjiang after one person was found to have the virus the previous day — the first new local cases for 10 days in mainland China. Even the poster child that is South Korea has confirmed 97 new cases of the coronavirus, a small uptick from the daily levels reported last week, just as officials ease social distancing restrictions after concluding that transmissions have slowed following a resurgence in mid-August.

In South America, Colombia became the eighth country to reach 1 million confirmed coronavirus cases. Two of the others are also in Latin America: Argentina, which hit that mark in the past week, and Brazil, which has more than 5 million confirmed cases.

Although these figures will be out of date very quickly, the trend is likely to remain for some time to come. All indicators point to this pandemic being far from over.

We know from experiences all over the world that no matter how good our defences, the virus can find a way through and we can find ourselves locked in a cycle of escalating case numbers all over again. Take Melbourne, Australia, which at the time of writing has just completed a 112-day second-wave lockdown (after recording zero new cases, four months earlier). The disruption that once seemed so novel and short term could continue for the foreseeable future and we may face further restrictions and localised lockdowns for months, or even years to come.

With the recognition that lockdown restrictions are likely to come and go again in the future, the excitement or fear you once felt at the announcement of the first lockdown may now have been replaced with a sense of dread, exhaustion, apathy or grim determination. It's difficult to return to restrictions when we've tasted freedom again. It's hard to summon the energy required to keep on keeping on when there is no natural conclusion in sight.

But there is the world as it is, and the world as we would like it to be. The world being as it is means that we're in this for the long haul. This is about adaptation to a future world with the coronavirus being present rather than a recovery to the world we knew in 2019. There is no 'new normal'. This phrase implies a static equilibrium, which is totally misleading because what we actually face is an ever-changing dynamic world where we are required to recalibrate, time and time again.

We know more about the virus than we did. Around the world, people are starting to engage with a pathway towards a more normal life, while trying to adapt public health measures to protect people while doing this. But then something happens and they are then perhaps catapulted back into further restrictions again. A careful balance has to be struck and it will look different in different places.

Rather than blaming individuals for failures of a system to protect us from the virus penetrating through various public health measures, we need to recognise that it is far more likely that there has been an unfortunate lining up of vulnerabilities in the system, meaning that the virus can slip through our best defences. Twenty years ago, James Reason called this the 'Swiss cheese model of system accidents'.

A systems approach to managing risk is to build layers of barriers and safeguards. In an ideal world, each barrier would be impenetrable, but in the real world there are likely to be vulnerabilities; like a slice of Swiss cheese, it has holes in it. So a hole in one layer caused by a mistake, a slip-up, fatigue or something else isn't necessarily catastrophic because there are other layers of defence to fall back on. And that all works fine unless all the layers have their holes lined up to form a channel through which your defences can be breached.

Wearing a mask, physical distancing, and washing your hands — three layers of defence that can reduce your risk of contracting Covid-19. But there's still a small chance that the virus can penetrate those layers and breach these defences. That's why wearing a mask has been added fairly late on in many countries. There was a growing realisation that added to a systems approach, it provides further protection, though it might not be all that effective by itself. However, combined with the other measures in place, it helps build up those layers and reduces the probability of a Swiss cheese type breach.

This is going to be choppy, there will be ups and down as the virus resurges from time to time, and we need to actively remind ourselves of what we need to do and how we need to act.

The dangers of complacency

As we've seen in chapter 12, one of the challenges of an ongoing public health crisis is stay-at-home or restriction fatigue. We start out with great intentions, but over time our enthusiasm and level of commitment to abiding by the rules wanes and that can push us into dangerous territory.

Let's take New Zealand as an example. Here, we were fortunate that the initial outbreak was small and caught early, and we were able to succeed in controlling the speed of the virus and eliminating community transmission during the initial lockdown period. At the time of writing, with most cases popping up at the border, or in managed isolation facilities, we need to be aware of the extreme dangers of complacency. There are worrying signs that this has already not so much crept in, as taken its seat at the head of the table. It's critical that we continue to remain vigilant, and behave in ways that protect us all.

For a moment, let's think of New Zealand as a person, and the borders of New Zealand as its skin. With a smooth skin, and no cuts or nicks, the border functions well to keep the coronavirus out. But where the skin ends — the nose, the mouth, the eyes, or where the skin gets cut — think of these like when border control breaks down, where people leave quarantine or managed isolation in unauthorised or uncontrolled ways. Well, that's when the virus can get into the body of New Zealand.

When this happens; if there is a suspected community outbreak, an 'immune system' response kicks in to identify and isolate the potential virus carriers, and then track back as many possible contacts as possible to determine whether they might also be a potential source of infection. If so, then the immune system quarantines those potential sources until either they are confirmed as a non-case or they become non-infectious.

In the meantime, we may need to protect the other parts of the 'body' of New Zealand by perhaps asking them to wear masks to both protect themselves and others from potential transmission and asking us to circulate less throughout the body of New

Zealand, limiting the risk of infected parts coming into contact with non-infected parts, and increasing the risk of spread. That would mean using tools like local, regional, or, in an extreme case, back to a national level lockdown. Or perhaps limiting movements into high-risk areas, like congregating together in numbers more than a few people, or returning to bubbles of safe contact. Nobody wants this, but it must remain part of our tools to change behaviour to limit the spread of the virus.

If we get underneath the skin, and see what's happening inside the body, then maybe it's interesting to think of the whole of New Zealand like a person who has recovered from a life-threatening health concern, e.g. a heart attack.

Once someone has been through the rehabilitation programme of watching what they eat, making sure they get appropriate exercise, and all the other things they are asked to do to reduce their risk of having another heart attack, many people manage to establish these as habits and go on to live healthy lives, continuing to manage their risk of further heart issues. They also participate in screening and wellness checks to make sure that all is well within their bodies.

Others find this more difficult and lapse back into old habits, and stop coming to appointments where they have medical tests to see how things are going, increasing their risk of another, possibly fatal, heart attack.

It's this reversion to past behaviour that we need to watch out for in terms of protecting ourselves and each other from Covid-19. Adopting new habits to keep checking in on our wellness before we get sick will be critical, so that means tracking your movements or using a Covid tracer app and taking a test and self-isolating if you develop symptoms. All this helps us to check on the state of the 'body' of New Zealand so we can get an early indication of when things might be going wrong, and so that we can mobilise our 'immune system' tools to control the outbreak as early as possible.

When thinking about another outbreak of Covid-19 in New Zealand spread through community transmission of the coronavirus, it's more a question of when rather than if. And at this point, we would do well to remember that aside from better technologies to detect the virus, the only tools we have are all based on behaviour.

How we behave now, as we work to prevent future outbreaks, and how we behave when these happen will be critical. Indeed, for the foreseeable future until safe, effective and widely accessible vaccines become available, they will most likely be the only tools we have.

Finding your compass in a Covid world

So how do we find our way forward in a Covid world? How can we hold on to a sense of optimism about the future and move forward in a meaningful way despite persistent uncertainty and change?

When we emerge from periods of lockdown and restriction, it can feel like we've just woken up and are blinking into the daylight, trying to let our eyes adjust and make sense of the world around us. While some of us may feel ready to run towards freedom, others might feel like they are letting go of the comfort of security and routine and moving into a place where things feel less predictable and certain than they were for the period of lockdown.

Take the time to understand that you might be going through a period of change — not just how the coronavirus might be changing the external world around us, but how it might be changing you too — even though you may never get infected by the virus itself.

Remember, we all have different experiences of these restrictions and different levels of tolerance for uncertainty, so this time may have impacted you in ways that it has not impacted your neighbour.

The other thing that's going on is a recalibration and realignment of the three systems of threat, calming and drive. When restrictions change, you need to figure out how to strike a new balance between your accelerator and your brake, and then activate your drive system to help you move forward. This is where you need a compass to help guide you through this uncharted territory in a way that's aligned with the way you want to live your life. And the best compass you have is your value system.

Your values steer your behaviour and your choices. Ever had that uneasy feeling in your stomach when you end up doing something at work or at home that doesn't sit well with you? That's your body telling you that you've behaved in a way that doesn't fit well with the values that you hold dear. Now you can ignore it and press on — which we sometimes have to do in the short term. Or we can reassess our behaviour so that it is in line with our values. Or we can sit down and figure out what our values are to give us a clue as to what we might want to do next.

Identifying your values will help you to recalibrate your life to the times. Coronavirus and uncertainty are going to be with us for a while to come, so now is the time to find your compass and become better at using it.

I don't want to minimise the difficult circumstances you may be facing right now, through no fault of your own. Getting your basic needs met will always be an important priority and the best predictor of how well people get through a crisis. But if you can develop some awareness and control over your reactions, how you want to navigate through the world and what is deeply important to you, then you may be able to direct yourself towards ways of being or doing that help your situation rather than making you feel even worse when the immediate life-threatening phase of the crisis has passed.

So how can you develop better awareness of your core values, and fine-tune how they steer you through these coronavirus times? Reflecting with our loved ones and close family and friends about our experiences in the first wave of the pandemic will help us prepare better for what comes next.

What did you emerge from lockdown appreciating more? What would you not like to leave in lockdown, but take with you into the next phase of life? This might give you a clue as to what may have changed for you.

For some, it was the ability to spend more time with kids and family in what might ordinarily be lives so busy that this didn't happen very often. For others, it might be the ability to understand and maybe change our attitudes about the dignity and worth of many occupations, such as bus drivers, cleaners and warehouse workers, as well as those working in health. Perhaps society has been forced to understand more clearly what work is 'key'. Perhaps you'll really remember people who enabled you to buy food for your families.

Lockdown experiences can also help to cultivate a sense of civic responsibility if people can connect personal sacrifices or discomfort to the broader public good to which we all contributed.

Maybe you're someone who values personal relationships, and closeness. Maybe you love the connection you feel when you're in a big crowd, maybe at a music festival. Maybe that is connecting to a sense of something bigger than you. And maybe we might have to find new ways of living in line with these closely held, or perhaps rediscovered, values. Or maybe there are revelations to you that only emerged after going through lockdown.

Recognise that this is a time of recalibration and realignment for many people. We know that people who go through disasters or emergencies often emerge on the other side with a new understanding and appreciation of what's important to them. They then start making changes in their lives so that the way they spend their time, who they work for, and the work they do feels more aligned to what drives them personally.

Of course, you may be in the position, like many, of taking whatever you can get to pay the bills. But your values also show up in how you deal with people, at work, and at home too.

Understanding, knowing and living by your compass or core values is one of the best ways to experience personal fulfilment and alignment with your inner truth — and not just in these pandemic times. Defining your personal core values will not only help you figure out what's truly important to you but also reduce anxiety and lead to making better decisions in your life.

Define your values

Here's an exercise for you to try to really zoom in on what drives you, and how it can help you to navigate some of the key decisions you need to make in times of crisis. Once you know your values, you can be sure to keep your sense of integrity and what you know is right for you, and approach decisions with confidence and clarity. You'll also know that what you're doing is best for your current and future happiness and satisfaction.

When you define your personal values, you discover what's truly important to you. A good way of starting to do this is to look back on your life — to identify when you felt really good, and really confident that you were making good choices.

Step 1: Identify the time you were happiest

Find examples from both your career and personal life, as this will ensure some balance in your answers. Ask yourself:

- What were you doing?
- Were you with other people? Who?
- What other factors contributed to your happiness?

Step 2: Identify the times you were most proud

- Use examples from your career and personal life. Why were you proud?
- Did other people share your pride? Who?
- What other factors contributed to your feelings of pride?

Step 3: Identify the times when you were most fulfilled and satisfied

Again, use both work and personal examples.

- What need or desire was fulfilled?

- How and why did the experience give your life meaning?
- What other factors contributed to your feelings of fulfilment?

Step 4: Choose your top values based on these experiences of happiness, pride and fulfilment

Why is each experience truly important and memorable for you? Use the following list of common personal values now that these experiences are topmost in your mind. Now that you're warmed up, it should make it easier than trying to pick out your values cold. Aim for about 10 values. And as you work through the list, you may find that some of these naturally combine. For instance, if you value philanthropy, community, and generosity, you might say that service to others is one of your top values.

Accountability	Excitement	Piety
Accuracy	Expertise	Positivity
Achievement	Exploration	Practicality
Adventurousness	Expressiveness	Preparedness
Altruism	Fairness	Professionalism
Ambition	Faith	Prudence
Assertiveness	Family-orientedness	Quality-orientation
Balance	Fidelity	Reliability
Being the best	Fitness	Resourcefulness
Belonging	Fluency	Restraint
Boldness	Focus	Results-oriented
Calmness	Freedom	Rigour
Carefulness	Fun	Security
Challenge	Generosity	Self-actualisation
Cheerfulness	Goodness	Self-control
Clear-mindedness	Grace	Selflessness
Commitment	Growth	Self-reliance
Community	Happiness	Sensitivity
Compassion	Hard work	Serenity
Competitiveness	Health	Service
Consistency	Helping society	Shrewdness
Contentment	Holiness	Simplicity
Continuous improvement	Honesty	Soundness
Contribution	Honour	Speed
Control	Humility	Spontaneity
Cooperation	Independence	Stability
Correctness	Ingenuity	Strategic
Courtesy	Inner harmony	Strength
Creativity	Inquisitiveness	Structure

Curiosity	Insightfulness	Success
Decisiveness	Intellectual status	Support
Democraticness	Intelligence	Teamwork
Dependability	Intuition	Temperance
Determination	Joy	Thankfulness
Devoutness	Justice	Thoroughness
Diligence	Leadership	Thoughtfulness
Discipline	Legacy	Timeliness
Discretion	Love	Tolerance
Diversity	Loyalty	Traditionalism
Dynamism	Making a difference	Trustworthiness
Economy	Mastery	Truth-seeking
Effectiveness	Merit	Understanding
Efficiency	Obedience	Uniqueness
Empathy	Openness	Unity
Enjoyment	Order	Usefulness
Enthusiasm	Originality	Vision
Equality	Patriotism	Vitality
Excellence	Perfection	

Step 5: For each of the 10 values you have now, ask yourself:

How important is that value to me on a scale of 1 to 10?

Now, pick your top three (and if there are more, narrow them down and keep grading them until you're left with only three).

Congratulations! You now have your top three values by which to guide your behaviour and decision-making. How do you do that? Well, the good news is that you don't need to wait for a pandemic or another crisis. The simplest answer is to incorporate everyday activities in accordance with your compass values.

If health is one of your top three values, ask yourself how can you live your life according to this value. Make healthy choices every single day: eat healthy food, have enough sleep, take care of your body and your mind.

Whatever your compass values are, chances are you weren't fully aware of them and that you neglect them on a day-to-day basis, just because you feel like you have too much on your plate. Use your compass values to guide you, and start to find your way to happiness, pride and a sense of fulfilment on a daily basis.

Developing self-regulation

Your values also play a role in self-regulation, which is an important attribute when it comes to maintaining the behaviours that keep us safe.

In simple terms, self-regulation is our ability to control our disruptive emotions, impulses and thoughts in the service of long-term goals. Self-regulation involves taking a pause between a feeling and an action — taking the time to think things through, make a plan, wait patiently. Children often struggle with these behaviours, and adults may as well.

People who self-regulate are also better able to see the good in other people, express themselves appropriately and see opportunities where others might not.

Self-regulation also enables you to act in accordance with your deeply held values or social conscience. If you value helping others, it will allow you to help a co-worker with a project, even if you are on a tight deadline yourself. It may also help you to stay at home or wear a mask to help stop any potential spread of coronavirus, or any other behaviours you're being asked to change for the greater good.

Your ability to self-regulate as an adult has roots in your development during childhood. In an ideal situation, a toddler who throws tantrums grows into a child who learns how to tolerate uncomfortable feelings without throwing a tantrum. Learning how to self-regulate as a child is an important skill for both emotional maturity and maintaining healthy social connections later on in life.

Parents can help develop self-regulation in children through routines, such as set mealtimes and set behaviours for each activity. Routines help children learn what to expect, which makes it easier for them to feel comfortable. When children act in ways that don't demonstrate self-regulation, parents can ignore their requests, such as making them wait if they interrupt a conversation. This works for us as adults too, which is why structure is so important.

As adults, the first step is to recognise that in every situation you have three options: approach, avoidance, and attack — or in other words, those threat system behaviours of fight, flight or freeze. While it may feel as though your choice of behaviour is out of your control, it's not. Your feelings may sway you more towards one path, but you are more than those feelings.

Bringing your values into play starts to calm your threat system down and bring your strategic brain back online as you start to focus on a wider range of behaviours that are available; more than those that are designed by your base evolutionary system to just keep you alive, but those behaviours that bring you those feelings of fulfilment, happiness and pride.

For example, if you find yourself wanting to break alert level restrictions, ask yourself these questions:

1. Is this what I really want to do?
2. Does this fit with my values?
3. How would I look at this behaviour in the future? How would I look at it if other people knew what I was doing?

The second step is to become aware of your transient feelings. For example, a rapidly increasing heart rate may be a sign that you are entering a state of irritation, rage or even a panic attack.

Start to restore balance by focusing on your deeply held values, rather than those transient emotions and bodily sensations. See beyond the discomfort of the moment to the larger picture. Then, act in a way that aligns with self-regulation.

By taking a moment to think about your compass values, you're building in that brake. Already your attention is starting to shift away from the threat. Your braking system then engages, as it detects your internal physiological system starting to shift away from the rapid heart rate and breathing. This signifies that the threat has passed and we can devote resources to other activities designed to help to adapt and thrive, rather than just survive on a moment-to-moment basis.

Remember, self-regulation involves taking a pause between a feeling and an action — taking the time to think things through, make a plan and wait patiently. These are vital attributes that will help you make good decisions and find your way forward in a Covid-19 world.

CHAPTER 14

What happens next?

As we grapple with our need to continue our lives when so much around us seems uncertain, we are discovering on a grand scale that being forced in and out of threat alert mode — on many different levels from individuals, to families, to communities to nations, and even the entire international community — does not make for the most optimal decision-making conditions.

So, besides a vaccine, what do we need most right now, and into the future, as what seemed like short-term solutions are being pivoted into ways of dealing with a longer-term threat?

Ironically, what we need most is the very opposite of what we are being pushed towards. It is also the thing that is most difficult to achieve in times of crisis and threat.

We are being pushed towards rigidity and denial. Some of our loved ones, and even some of our key decision-makers and leaders, may be afraid. Their coping strategy to reduce their anxiety is downplay the crisis, rather than face what is real and unrelenting. The danger is that they will hold fast to the narrative that there is nothing to be concerned about, bolstered by one of the cognitive biases we may be prone to when feeling under threat and stress. And when they do make decisions, they will make them far too late.

This particular bias has been called the 'Status quo bias'. It refers to people's preference for a sense of familiarity and for things to stay as they are, with inertia taking priority over action. This may in part explain why some governments were more willing to accept the status quo and ignore warnings of the devastating consequences of pandemics, even though the need for pandemic preparedness had been clearly and repeatedly stated.

Related to this is a tight clinging to old habits, especially those driven by self-interest, where members of the public, and even senior figures in public life, have given in to the temptation to ignore physical distancing guidance and have ventured out, or have ignored advice to wear a mask while doing so. I'll name no names here but I'm sure you know some examples in your own locality.

What we most need, the most valuable attitude and asset we can have, is **flexibility**. A cognitive flexibility enabling us to hold ideas lightly, and to change behaviour rapidly in the face of changing circumstances or new information. And an emotional flexibility that enables us to manage these changes in behaviour without dropping into threat states of mind, or the rigidity in thinking and behaviour which plunges us back into denial of reality and wishful thinking.

Unfortunately, flexibility is also one of the hardest things to access in times of uncertainty. Aside from the physical threat of the coronavirus itself, the looming threat of its resurgence means that maintaining and managing the optimal social and mental conditions for flexibility is likely to be the single most enormous challenge that we will have to manage in these pandemic times.

Facing this particular brand of uncertainty is hard. The ground seems to be constantly shifting beneath you as you try to come to terms with being in and out of various states of limbo. There's no firm endpoint in sight, and the usual settings of your life are largely disrupted.

Tie this to our usual craving for predictability and routine, and it's no surprise that we often find uncertainty more difficult to handle than definitively knowing something bad is going to happen. And that's why in the middle of this it's so important to remind ourselves that uncertainty regarding this pandemic will not last for ever. We can and will make it through, together.

It's important to acknowledge the things you've lost and made sacrifices for during the pandemic, with its associated limits, disruptions and lockdowns. These are all significant. It's okay and you have every right to feel grief for the quick goodbyes to friends and family, uncertainty about when you'll see each other again, missed celebrations for birthdays and anniversaries. In fact, mourning can be healthy as you name your grief and face it head-on, rather than pushing it aside as if nothing has happened.

The grief you may be experiencing may involve feelings of loss about your sense of belonging. You may no longer have all the people around you on a day-to-day basis that make up your community and you may find yourself wondering where you fit in now. A feeling of loss of place may show itself if you miss your workplace, your college, your school, or the places you used to hang out. You may acutely feel a loss of independence if you suddenly have to head back to your family home for the first time in years, or perhaps to some other living arrangement instead of what you have become used to. And then there is a loss of a sense of wellbeing, perhaps amplified by economic difficulties, uncertainties about employment, changes in your educational arrangements and loss of anticipated gatherings and celebrations. All this can leave us feeling deeply unsettled, uneasy, and even traumatised.

This loss of wellbeing was real, as reported is the latest research here in New Zealand.[1] While New Zealand's lockdown successfully

1. Every-Palmer, S, Jenkins, M, Gendall, P, Hoek, J, Beaglehole, B, Bell, C, Williman, J, Rapsey, C & Stanley, J (2020). Psychological distress, anxiety, family violence,

eliminated Covid-19 from the community, the achievement took a psychological toll, with almost one-third experiencing moderate to severe psychological distress and one in 10 reporting some form of family harm during alert level 4, the most stringent lockdown level.

Add to this the sense of anticipatory grief that we may have been feeling for a while now: our concerns about the future and what it holds when we're surrounded by uncertainty. And to compound it all, add ambiguous loss — things that have not yet taken shape in our lives but involves lost dreams, imagined futures, the feeling of stable safety that so many of us used to have in our lives, as well as the sense of living in a stable world, rather than this constantly shifting parallel universe we can sometimes feel like we have been teleported to, where we can feel safe one minute, and be thrown into despair the next.

Take a moment to realise that all the accumulated losses are significant. Give yourself the time and space to grieve, to cry, to be fearful, and to feel like life is unfair. Let out the sadness and the anger, and comfort one another, and talk about what you are mourning. There is power in language. There is power in pausing to reflect. There is power in realising what we have lost so that we can eventually emerge from this grief to take our next steps.

The anxiety that rises up from time to time and threatens to drown us in its depths can feel terrifying. It is so important to keep in mind that this time of pandemic and worry isn't permanent. But that is much easier said than done.

As well as individual ways to manage anxiety that I've discussed

suicidality, and wellbeing in New Zealand during the COVID-19 lockdown: A cross-sectional study. PLOS ONE. Published 4 November 2020, https://doi.org/10.1371/journal.pone.0241658

in this book, recognise that anxiety can sometimes be contagious. So, try not to constantly discuss the pandemic and its impacts with others where you feed each other's anxieties. You might also be susceptible to empathic stress, where you take on some emotions that others are feeling during challenging times. This makes having coping mechanisms that are healthy for you even more important at this time. I know that this is something that I have to work particularly hard on.

To engage the calming system rapidly, try the 5-4-3-2-1 exercise, where you ground yourself by identifying five things you can see around you, four things you can touch, three things you can hear, two things you can smell, and one thing you can taste. Be sure to take long, slow, deep breaths to enhance the calm. Remember, your Default Mode Network in your brain does not function so actively when you are paying attention to your senses. So all the catastrophic thoughts and worries associated with activation of the Default Network, the ones that create nightmare scenarios in your mind when you're doom-scrolling on your cellphone, don't have room to take hold when you're paying attention to your senses in this way. If this is a problem for you, make it a regular habit to manage your anxiety through paying particular attention to your senses.

A specific form of emotional challenge that is taking shape for many people who are temporarily isolated from the people and life that they knew is known as isolation anxiety. Once you add in the uncertainty and the mourning of lost opportunities like long-distance or overseas travel to see family and friends, there is a potential that this may feel potentially overwhelming for some.

Isolation can exacerbate existing mental health conditions, so it's important to stick with medication, self-care and counselling if this is what has worked for us in the past. But to prepare for longer terms of separation from the lives we used to know, we may need to build daily ways into helping us to prevent an isolation spiral. This might include:

- **Turn physical distancing to social cohesion.** When in periods of lockdown or shutdown, connect with your people in all the technological and from-afar ways that you know how.
- **Find things to do.** Do one productive thing in your immediate surroundings each day, from personal projects to helping a neighbour safely. This way, you can feel less 'stuck' and more accomplished.
- **Stick as close to your routine as possible.** This will help you to stay as active and engaged as possible, instead of lethargic and unmotivated. It's an easy thing to fall out of routine, so if you do, don't be too hard on yourself, and start again the next day. Keeping your routines — even though they may look a little different to before the pandemic struck — will make it easier to adjust when the period of isolation ends.
- **Help others safely.** Become more externally focused to get outside your own internal struggle. Check on others, send positive messages, engage in local efforts and reach out.
- **Don't obsess over endless pandemic coverage.** Don't skew your perspective and increase your anxiety by googling every possible symptom, or spend too much time being served what the social media algorithms are predicting you're going to click on — even if you know it'll probably make you feel worse than you already do. Or even worse, amplify feelings of anger and separation with the danger of deepening your sense of unfairness that is actually far removed from reality. Limit your media consumption and only tap into reliable sources of information.
- **Start new rituals.** Give yourself something to look forward to, whether it's a regular video chat with friends, safe walks,

journaling or playing games with family over the internet. It will help you feel like you're making the most of this time rather than seeing everything as a lost opportunity.

There's been no other global collective experience like this pandemic that has demanded new levels of psychological flexibility from so many of us, all at the same time. Whether we like it or not, we are being asked to bend, flex and adapt in ways we never knew were possible — indeed, in many ways which were previously thought to be flat-out impossible.

There are certain things we do actually need to be concrete about, like making sure we wash our hands, staying away from large gatherings and practising physical distancing. And in terms of broader preparedness, making sure we have access to water and also stocking the cupboards with dry goods for unexpected lockdowns — though this is easier said than done for many feeling the economic pressure in these pandemic times.

What I'm talking about here is different. Having psychological flexibility is to have the ability to shift perspectives and actions when new or unexpected events come up. The more flexible we can be, the more we can adapt to meet otherwise stressful and difficult situations and changes without becoming overwhelmed for long periods of time.

We already use these skills of psychological flexibility in our daily lives when we manage last-minute schedule changes, having to work at home when a child is ill, or making decisions about what we can or can't do when weekend plans change. What's new is millions of people having to practise increased psychological flexibility all at the same time, when whole cities, and indeed whole countries, go into lockdown.

As the coronavirus pulses in its distribution around the world, and as countries flex their public health measures and requests for people to limit their contact with each other and to restrict their movements, then we will be called upon to respond to these pulses or pandemic policy pivot in how governments react in ways that require psychological flexibility and clear thinking.

Maintaining and improving a psychologically flexible mindset will be a crucial skill to hone and practise for us to think clearly and thoroughly; because this is the only alternative to falling into chronic despair, despondency, simply tuning out, and anxiety. Alternatively, there lies the path of denial with angry lashing out against all that disagree with the narratives of denial, and the conspiracy theories and the societal divisions that may accompany that.

To stay flexible in times of fear is difficult, and people will often retreat into survival mode, resulting in rigidity, holding tightly to 'tried and true' behaviours in response to frightening situations. But psychological flexibility can be practised and improved. And there is no time when it has been needed more.

In order to successfully navigate these pandemic times, here is the radical acceptance leap we need to make:

1. **Remind yourself** that what you are feeling — the fear, the anxiety — is normal. It's okay to feel that way.
2. **Reality is what it is.** The facts about the present are the facts, even if you don't like them.
3. **This is more about adaptation to a future with the coronavirus being present**, rather than eradicating it as a threat.
4. **There are limitations on the future for everyone,** but we still have choices about what limitations we want to accept.
5. **Life can be worth living well,** even with painful events in it.

6. **Pain is likely,** but it doesn't have to lead to unending suffering.

What can we do when the pain of fear, anxiety, and grief arises? We actually need to feel the emotion, and resist the temptation to suppress it and deny that it is happening.

1. **Name the emotion.** It seems true that if we can name the emotion, that is the first step in helping to 'tame' it. It's why we spend so much time helping children to name what they are feeling.
2. **Acknowledge that all emotions are okay.** They have emerged for a reason. If we pay attention to them, we can recognise the clues to help us figure out what we need.
3. **Talk about your emotions** with people who can hold them with you, with support and empathy. This can be friends, family, or professional help.
4. **Recognise that we are not alone** in our pain and suffering, and be as kind to yourself as you would be to a loved one. Noticing our shared humanity is an important step towards being more compassionate with ourselves.

The road to a resolution of our pandemic journey will be a long one. Things will be different once we get there. We will be different once we get there. And we will, if we can look after each other with care and ourselves with self-compassion.

This is the reality that will be hard for us to accept. Instead of denial and rigidity, what we actually need is flexibility and compassion: a recognition of our common humanity. When we can intentionally exercise our ability to switch down the threat state of our minds, and to unlock the flexibility that comes with practices that generate calm, only then will we be able to fully appreciate the joys of living when they arise in these pandemic times.

It is worth noting that in the recent New Zealand research,[2] almost 40% reported low wellbeing and about one third reported moderate-to-high distress, but over 60% of people also experienced 'silver linings' at alert level 4, such as more time with family.

Make no mistake, there are stormy times ahead. Some days it will be bright blue sky and calm seas, but other days, it will be rough weather. Some people will feel unsettled more than others, and sometimes you'll feel more unsettled. Reach out, be strong when you can, but it's okay to need help and be vulnerable too.

Finally, you might be wondering what meaning we will find in all this. Some people, and I agree with them, believe we will find light in these times. Even now people are realising they can connect through technology and are not as remote or as isolated as they once thought. They are picking up the phone again and having long conversations. They are appreciating walks in the sunshine, school teachers and the ability to explore close to home. I believe we will continue to find new layers of meaning as our Covid-19 journey progresses.

This book came about as I sensed a need to share what I have learned through a thirty-year career as a psychologist, and being deeply involved in emergency management and understanding how to help others going through disaster, emergency and crisis in the past 14 years. One of my most vivid memories through the last

2. Every-Palmer, S, Jenkins, M, Gendall, P, Hoek, J, Beaglehole, B, Bell, C, Williman, J, Rapsey, C & Stanley, J (2020). Psychological distress, anxiety, family violence, suicidality, and wellbeing in New Zealand during the COVID-19 lockdown: A cross-sectional study. PLOS ONE. Published 4 November 2020, https://doi.org/10.1371/journal.pone.0241658

few months was turning up at the advertising agency tasked with building the New Zealand Government's 'Unite Against Covid-19' campaign, in March 2020, just as we were about to enter level 4 lockdown, with two words in mind: structure and empathy. Mark Dalton, the Creative Director at the agency, recently commented that he found this conversation helpful, and it seems as though the word empathy resonated especially with him:

> 'Dr Sarb Johal, who had done a lot of prior work on the H1N1 influenza outbreak in the UK, and then helping communities in New Zealand recover from earthquakes, has been really helpful to us. He says that the most important thing you can do is have empathy. Whatever you do, you must try to be empathetic and helpful in your design work and the language you put into it. All people really want to know is what's the right thing to do, whether they're doing it, and if it is working.'[3]

I hope this book helps you to uncover a little more empathy and structure, for yourselves, and each other, as we continue to travel through these challenging and difficult times. Together.

3. https://www.wallpaper.com/design/mark-dalton-design-helping-people-through-pandemic-by-design

Afterword

As I write this in January 2021, new variants of the virus have emerged in both the UK and South Africa. Because of their more transmissible nature — around 50 to 70% more contagious — these variants are expected to become more common over the world over the next few months. And when outbreaks take place, they will become more difficult to contain, requiring more demanding controls, lasting for longer periods of time. These may not be the only new variants we have to deal with.

Even with vaccines remaining effective and now becoming more accessible, the logistics of maintaining transport and cold storage supply chains, and having enough people to inject others is challenging.

I'm optimistic that we will emerge from this. But I am also realistic enough to realise that we have a hard road ahead, as we see waves of infection emerge and gather pace across borders and continents.

I have seen estimates that we will see a return to normal life by Easter 2021. I have my doubts. There will be moments of hope, like when we see further vaccines come online. But they will be coupled to deeply challenging times, such as in the UK right now where, as I write, a new lockdown has commenced lasting for at least six weeks.

Clarity through coordinated and coherent communication will be even more crucial than it has been so far, across local, regional governments, and at the level of national governments too. Even at a time where geopolitics are fraught and nationalism and protectionism have come to the fore, international cooperation can still make a big difference to how this pandemic will play out across the world. However, this relies on a shared determination to make this happen, and wise leadership emerging from the turmoil.

Difficult debates will continue and additional issues will emerge as we spend extended periods of time in these altered states of social contact and economic activity. For example:

- The threat to mental health has been used as an argument against lockdowns. But there are good mental health arguments for controlling the virus too. As well as the fear of becoming infected or having vulnerable loved ones fall ill, suffering severe disease can exacerbate mental health problems, or trigger new ones. Are we getting this balance right?
- More people are likely to come forward for help with moderate to severe mental health issues — people who have never experienced issues before. How do we re-configure services and help to meet this need?
- Where face-to-face meetings are discouraged, and even getting a video consultation for counselling is difficult, how do we manage the large increases in prescribing antidepressants, and the consequences of this?
- How do we prepare teachers for a significant number of children entering and progressing through the education system who have not only had less social interaction with other children and adults, but have also spent much of that time seeing faces partially covered up with masks? How might their recognition of emotions and their own emotional regulation be affected by these and other factors, and how can we assist their ongoing development?

There is no new normal.

There is only change.

And this can be difficult to accept.

We must accept and tackle these emerging issues with a calm and deliberative focus, rather than knee-jerk responses designed to deal with immediate threats rather than understanding the wider context. Leaders must not become preoccupied with saving face or avoiding tough decisions in order to avoid unpopularity, which is another way that our threat detection system leads us to make poor decisions.

Clear, coherent, consistent, and strategic action and communication are needed now more than ever to avoid prolonging the struggles of many people living through these times.

And we can only do this when we are calm.

About the Author

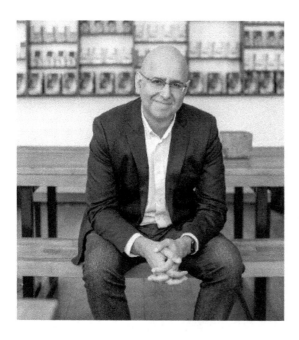

Born in the UK where he trained as a Clinical Psychologist, Dr Sarb Johal's experience encompasses clinical practice, frontline services, policy development and Ministerial advice and strategic communications.

Since 2006, he has helped the New Zealand and UK governments, as well as the World Health Organisation, develop psychosocial responses to some of the major crises of the last decade, including the H1N1 pandemic, the Canterbury earthquakes, the Kaikōura earthquake, the Christchurch mosque shootings and most recently, the Covid-19 pandemic. Dr Johal lives in Wellington with his wife and young family.

https://sarbjohal.com/

Acknowledgements

I remember going into the kitchen one evening back in March, and I said to my wife that I think this is going to get really intense, and that if I started to lose my way, I wanted her to remind me that I was to stick to talking about structure and empathy, even though everything might get really complicated.

These were my navigation points.

I know I wouldn't have been able to write this book, and indeed do any of my work, without the support of my wonderful wife, Sarah Johal. The fact that I get to live with you and see you every day never ceases to amaze me how lucky I have been to find you. And you make amazing cheese scones. This is me letting the rest of the world know: this book became a reality because of you.

You are my compass.

Thank you to our daughters, Liv, Daia, and Sianna — thank you for the fantastic dancing interludes, and incessant kids TV and music videos that sparked crazy ideas in my mind for videos and book sections.

You are my anchors.

Taking our dog Benji out for walks has been brilliant for me in the mornings as an opportunity for me to get out of my own head, even if just for a few minutes. And even our antisocial cat Ruru had her moments of empathy during particularly intense times over the past few months.

It's been so hard to be apart from my parents during this time. This has been the longest period of time that I have been physically apart from them, and I know it's been particularly difficult for them too, as older adults who remain in London, where they emigrated to in the 1960s, and where I was born, raised and later completed my clinical training. They have been so supportive of the very unconventional career zigzags I have taken, sometimes bemused but always 100% behind me. And I am so thankful and grateful for their support and guidance. It is really only recently that they have talked about their own difficult early years, and how they became refugees after the partition of India. I hope to see them soon again back in London.

I miss you.

None of this journey should be undertaken alone, even if we are being asked to be physically distant at times right now. As well as those I've already mentioned, Lori Satterthwaite and Christine Sheehy have been great in my team in helping me to get my website and this book together, as well as all the people in the New Zealand media and the Science Media Centre with whom I have worked with so often in 2020.

Take care out there.

Sarb Johal
December 2020
Wellington, New Zealand

— Notes —

Notes